Skeletons Without Bones

Dragging Recovered Memories of
Sexual Abuse Out of the Closet

Skeletons Without Bones

Donna McGraw Laurence & Rosalyn J. Titus

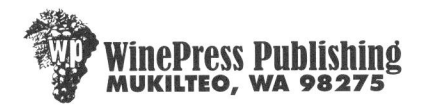

WinePress Publishing
MUKILTEO, WA 98275

Skeletons Without Bones
Copyright © 1998 Donna McGraw Laurence & Rosalyn J. Titus

Published by:
WinePress Publishing
PO Box 1406
Mukilteo, WA 98275

All rights reserved. No part of this publication may be reproduced, stored in a retrieval system or transmitted in any way by any means, electronic, mechanical, photocopy, recording or otherwise, without the prior permission of the publisher, except as provided by USA copyright law.

Scripture is quoted from the King James Version of the Bible.

Printed in the United States of America

ISBN 1-57921-077-5
Library of Congress Catalog Card Number: 97-62306

Contents

Acknowledgements vii
Foreword ix
Introduction xi

Chapter One—Initiation 13

Chapter Two—"I Wish You Had Known My Daddy" 23

Chapter Three—In the Viper's Den 35

Chapter Four—Dr. French: Friend or Fraud? 49

Chapter Five—Aftermath 61

Chapter Six—To the Accuser Belong the Spoils 67

Chapter Seven—"In the Mouth of Two or Three Witnesses" . . 77

Chapter Eight—The Man I Call Daddy! 83

Chapter Nine—Hanging Out the Dirty Laundry 101

Chapter Ten—"Her Children . . . Call Her Blessed" 107

Chapter Eleven—Documenting the Past 121

Chapter Twelve—Westward Ho! 127

Chapter Thirteen—Therapist or The*RAPIST*? 129

Chapter Fourteen—"Unto the Third . . . Generation" 143

Chapter Fifteen—The Elephant in the Living Room 153

Chapter Sixteen—The Family Fights Back 159

Chapter Seventeen—A Declaration of Defense 165

Chapter Eighteen—Trapped in the Trappings 171

Chapter Nineteen—Beware! Epidemic! 195

Chapter Twenty—The Turning of the Tide 201

Chapter Twenty-One—If an Accusation Is Made 213

Epilogue—Why This Book? 221
Notes 225
Bibliography 231

Acknowledgements

There is no adequate way to thank the many people who helped, in one way or another, produce this book. I am deeply indebted to them all.

Son Dustin insisted there was a story begging to be told. Niece Rose stood by, pen in hand. Sister-in-law Kay laboriously transcribed tapes and did research.

My husband Gary became secretary and word processor, as well as my encourager and greatest fan. I couldn't have done it without him, nor would I want to.

Pauline Phillippe and Janet May have been in my corner over the long haul, their faith in me never wavering.

Marion Cozby and Barb Armstrong enthused over the early chapters. Dr. Wayne Caldwell and Dr. Elizabeth Loftus gave of their time to encourage me along. Several *former* friends dared to critique my work and offer suggestions.

Family members helped in numerous ways, even those who at first were dubious about the project. Nieces Danita and Shannon proved to me the effort was worth it.

Sharon Bridwell gave invaluable insight and suggestions. Etta Miller proofread and helped hone the finished manuscript.

I am also grateful to the legion of editors who sent rejection slips, forcing me to self-publish; to Donna Dightman who lured me to a seminar about self-publishing; and to Athena Dean who took an interest in a manuscript dubbed "Big Red."

Absolutely no credit goes to my clone, Linda Beveridge, who has continued to remain uninterested in my literary efforts. She should have paid attention because she will doubtless be blamed for writing this book. I expect she will sign autographs without so much as batting an eye.

Foreword

Truth is stranger than fiction. But when fiction, garbed in academic robes, supplants truth, it is worse than strange; it is tragic.

This book is, to my best knowledge, a true account of events that happened within my family. With the exception of Dad, who died in 1984, and Mother, who as I write this is in a nursing home, my relatives portrayed herein are alive and well as the book goes to press.

The question often put to me is some variation of, "What do the members of your family think about your writing this book?" I understand and appreciate the concern expressed by the query. It is one that I, too, pondered as I worked on the manuscript. For that reason I used all fictitious names, changing them to actual names only if the person referenced gave me permission to do so.

Thankfully, this book has functioned as a catalyst to bring restoration within my family. First, it forced us to acknowledge "the elephant in the living room." Second, it equipped each of us with the knowledge necessary to make informed decisions as to what we should do about its presence.

The result? The exposure has revealed the beast as the paper tiger—er, elephant—that it was, and it has been subsequently discarded. The elephant no longer occupies our front room.

A letter from my sister Anna dated October 19, 1997, fairly well summarizes—with one obvious exception—the sentiments of my family:

> Reading and discussing the book gave me a whole different perspective on everything. I began to see I had been believing a bunch of lies. I began to comprehend how you had felt. I understand that the book had to be written. In my opinion it is a perfect blend of truth, humor, pain, sorrow, tragedy, instruction, fun, sarcasm, and Christian testimony.

The exception would be Lillian. Two years ago I gave her a copy of the manuscript and asked that she read it. I do not know if she has done so.

I do know this, however. If Lillian still entertains the elephant, she entertains it alone.

Introduction

When the wizardry of therapy, aided by drugs and hypnosis, unearths a land mine of long-buried memories of sexual abuse, the detonation of such a discovery ravages an entire family. Cut down without warning from within the sanctuary of "Home, Sweet Home," family members have no time to seek cover, no means of self-defense and no way of escape. The accused, who is assumed guilty until proven innocent, is catapulted into a most preposterous position. He is compelled either to admit guilt, or else he must prove he did not commit a crime in seclusion some years, or even decades, before.

No one denies that abuse is rampant throughout our culture. When it has in fact occurred, it has been done in secret, without the presence of witnesses, thereby making it most difficult to establish guilt.

However, in cases where the alleged abuse has *not* occurred, there can *never* be witnesses to a non-event, thereby making it *impossible* to verify innocence.

Unable to prove the unprovable, the accused suddenly discovers his reputation ruined, his mind fragmented and his family in disarray. Often his life, his health, his finances and his marriage all lie in ruins. He may spend the rest of his life ostracized by loved ones and acquaintances. Quite possibly he may end up behind bars.

Meanwhile, the fabricators of the abuse, i.e., the accuser and the counselor, both may enjoy clemency, financial compensation, public affirmation and celebrity status, complete with glitzy media coverage. If the accuser/counselor team has been exceptionally creative in constructing "memories," they may be rewarded with a best-selling book and a box office hit.

We, the authors of **Skeletons Without Bones**, are descendants of one such unjustly accused man. His mind disoriented by the erosion of Alzheimer's disease, our father (and grandfather) could scarcely tell you his name. How could he defend himself against a clandestine kangaroo court operating out of a psychologist's office thousands of miles away? Even men with all their faculties intact are seldom able to exonerate themselves when faced with an array of experts who assume the guilt of the accused *without a shred of evidence.*

Daddy went to his grave with his name maligned, without recourse and without justice. At the time of this writing, his widow still lives under the shadow of those unfounded stories.

Speaking for ourselves and on behalf of thousands of suffering families, we contend the time has come to expose and expunge these privileged guerrillas and their terrorist tactics. We declare that truth must be granted its day in court. We protest that *real* memories can be recalled without psychological hocus-pocus. We *insist* that *real* skeletons have bones.

We do not act under concealment provided by closed doors, drawn curtains, darkened rooms and selected audiences. Instead, we unlock the doors, throw open the windows and turn on the lights. We invite the world to investigate, deliberate, and draw intelligent conclusions.

We stand confident that virtue shines all the more brightly when scrutinized under the unbiased searchlight of truth.

CHAPTER ONE

Initiation

Anticipation threatened to succumb to panic as I squirmed in the passenger seat of my sister Ginny's[1] car. With each mile, the impending confrontation loomed closer and closer, filling me with dread. But after years of veiled insinuations, outright attacks and indignant defenses transmitted over the family grapevine, we remained mired in a hopeless impasse. Now I was about to participate in an encounter which I hoped would lead us to resolution.

As we traveled those forty-five miles to our point of rendezvous, suspense heightened as when one watches a spell-binding TV mystery. Whatever lurks behind that closed door threatens to be dreadful, but you watch in fascinated horror, ready to dismember anyone who would dare switch the channel!

The difference, of course, was that this drama was not composed of movie stars playing roles. The cast consisted of members of my own family, with the glaring exception of one guest star. Adrenalin surged as I prepared to make my debut, entering center stage—without having seen the script.

Driving between cities in the great Northwest where Ginny had made her home for over a decade, we were headed for the office of her psychologist and mentor of almost as many years. There we would meet our younger sister Lillian, also a long-standing client of the same counselor.

I hoped I was not a "fool rushing in" as I ventured onto turf belonging to these two sisters. When Lillian had remarked to her therapist, "I wish I could tell Donna," he had encouraged her to make her wish come true. So here I was, about to be made privy to the dark secret that lay heavy in the bosom of our fractured family.

Only to those two sisters did this mystery possess form and substance enough to qualify as a *bona fide* secret. To the rest of us, it more resembled a mysterious shadow enshrouding us in an impenetrable darkness. For years it had remained an unnameable, irrational, unwelcome intrusion, refusing to assume a shape we could identify or a form with which we could wrestle.

The prospect of ferreting out our shadowy foe had produced in me this dreadful anticipation. I hoped that once the adversary had been identified and forced out of hiding, we could openly grapple with it and overthrow its tyrannical hold on our family.

I did not share my sisters' high esteem for their psychologist, John George French. Although most of the family, myself included, had not been told the nature of Lillian's problem, nor did we understand Ginny's less serious hang-ups, we had been inundated with reports describing their wonderful counselor. To Ginny and Lillian he possessed divine-like qualities.

From what we had heard of him and from reading material he had written or recommended, some of us considered him an impostor, a fraud, and a colossal opportunist. Having met him on several occasions, I detested his condescending attitude. I am certain he was equally uncharmed by me.

Expediency forced me to set aside my personal feelings in deference to this unprecedented occasion. Except for her interaction with Ginny and my oldest sister Anna and their children, Lillian had cut herself off from all other family contacts. We who lived in other parts of the country had been warned by the great doctor as to how we were to conduct ourselves in the event we were allowed a brief encounter with her.

Now Lillian wanted to risk opening up to one of the uninitiated, albeit in the presence of her therapist. So here I was, hoping to discover the cause of Lillian's personal disintegration and her alienation from her family.

Yes, things were changing, and I responded with a mixture of fear and relief. But I was ready. Come what may, I was ready.

Dr. French's office occupied one wing of his spacious home, recently constructed in the picturesque rural setting which spread out around us. His horses watched blandly from beyond the fence as we parked the car and entered the empty waiting room. Lillian and Dr. French must have been sequestered somewhere beyond the closed office door.

Ginny made herself comfortable with a book, preparing to sit this one out. No doubt I was expected to do the same while I awaited my summons. Glancing around the room to review my options, I spied a folded piece of paper lying on the arm of the sofa. Seeing my name written in Lillian's handwriting, I wondered why a note would precede a scheduled conversation. I hoped she hadn't changed her mind because—well, because I was here, and I was ready.

Unfolding the paper, I instantly discerned its horrific contents. Numbed and stupefied, my eyes stared at what my brain could not conceive.

And I knew—I was *not* ready.

My father was a clergyman who for many years had pastored small town or rural churches in America's heartland. Since additional income was necessary to supplement the earnings supplied by his small congregations, Dad usually held an additional full time job. Mom stood by his side, the embodiment of the title "Mother," spending her time and herself rearing twelve children and mothering many more.

Skeletons Without Bones

Our household never knew an abundance of money, but we were abundantly rich. We made our own fun doing simple things together. In addition to our own perpetual supply of resident teenagers, neighborhood kids gravitated to our house just to hang out, adding hilarity to pure mayhem.

In spite of already bulging walls, for years our basement was designated bachelor quarters for half-a-dozen recent high school graduates who came from surrounding towns to find employment at our church's international headquarters in Syracuse, New York, where my father worked. Weekends these boys migrated home, often taking some of us kids from their adopted family to visit their real families.

During the week they ate supper with us and participated in our evening activities. Our dining room table, its extra leaves permanently installed, daily accommodated anywhere from twelve to more-than-twenty hungry diners.

Our house boasted no dishwasher, no TV, no stereo, and only one bathroom. But it produced plenty of serious debates, lively conversations, games of dominoes, Monopoly[2] or "kick the can," and some fine harmonizing sessions around the piano—perhaps all the above happening at the same time—providing ample entertainment for everyone.

Through it all, Mother and Daddy maintained their equilibrium, never quarreling or cutting each other down. They worked hard without losing their ability to laugh. I often saw them weary; I never saw them out of sorts.

Some Saturday mornings Dad would take over the kitchen, producing his wonderful deep-dish pies—apple, peach or berry—or his famous pumpkin or chocolate creations. Wintery Saturday nights often would find him whipping up an immense batch of candy, setting huge platters full of rich, dark fudge to cool and harden in the snow on the back porch. But more often his Saturday night routine included polishing six to eight pairs of shoes and setting them in a neat, shiny row, ready to be worn to Sunday school the next morning. Mother, meanwhile, presided over the

Saturday night bath and shampoo routine, making sure we kids shone as brightly as our footwear.

A move from New York State to Indiana did not alter the neighborhood hangout status of our house. Recently my friend Vicki reminisced how she enjoyed being included within the circle of our boisterous family. "I was always welcome to Sunday dinner at your house, except when you had pork chops." Dad, who did most of the grocery shopping, brought home one pork chop per person—no more, no less. We kids learned to be frugal, if not downright stingy, with our rations. Rather than give up such a prized morsel, we avoided bringing guests home on a pork chop Sunday.

But more often, pot roast or fried chicken graced our Sunday table. Mother insisted her favorite poultry pieces were the backs and necks. I now realize that once the platter had circled our stretched-out table, she was indeed fortunate if there remained anything but bony pieces for her to choose.

During those years we produced skyscrapers of dirty dishes and mountains of laundry. Late at night Mother could often be found seated on the sofa, sound asleep, with neat piles of folded clothes all around her.

Years later, at the time Ginny and I commenced upon our momentous journey, that teeming household had given way to one that moved at a more sedate pace. Now in their retirement years, my folks resided in Puerto Rico where they kept the home fires burning for granddaughter Esther Ruth, a student at the Conservatory of Music in Rio Piedras. Esther's parents, Bill and Millie Goldsmith, had left their missionary assignment in Puerto Rico to begin a new work in Santo Domingo.

Although Daddy was fighting a losing battle with Alzheimer's disease, for two years my parents enjoyed a reciprocal love affair with the Puerto Rican parishioners who delighted in watching over them and spoiling them. In return, the church community thrived on Mother's nurturing and witnessed the wonder of my parents' continued devotion to one another during Daddy's mental deterioration.

Skeletons Without Bones

Back in Dr. French's waiting room, numbed in body and mind, I gaped stupidly at my sister's handwritten message:

> *Donna, When I was a little girl Daddy repeatedly sexually molested me. I was very little—3 or 4 or 5 I think. He would take me back in the room behind the platform in Baldwinsville where he studied. He would hold the* Radio Talks[3] *book in one hand while he read it to me. With his other hand he would rub my stomach. Then he would pick up another book and give it to me to hold. It had a soft, silky cover. He would say, "Lillian's tummy is soft and smooth like the pretty book." His hand would reach down into my panties. Then he would put me down and angrily tell me to take off all my clothes. Then he would angrily say, "You are a naughty, nasty little girl. Look at you, standing there with your clothes off. Look at yourself! God has given Daddies special ways to punish naughty little girls." He would tell me to get up and lay down on the cot. Then he would molest me, it was rectal and oral, I think. Then he would go back to his desk and read. After a while he would turn around and say, no longer angrily, "Lillian, why do you have your clothes off? Put them back on." So I would get dressed. Sometimes he would tell me nothing happened. That I had had a bad, naughty dream, or that I had imagined it. And I mustn't tell anyone I had those kinds of thoughts or dreams. Sometimes he would say, "Now you won't be bad like your mother." It happened over and over again, over a period of time, I don't know how long.*

The letter ended as abruptly as it had begun.
No—*most emphatically NO!*—I was *not* ready!

Nothing in my nearly forty years had prepared me for the contents of that note. In my most off-the-wall conjecturing, I could not have dredged up the obscenity scrawled dogmatically across that page, now etched irrevocably on my recoiling mind.

Dr. French confiscated that note addressed to me, "to place it in Lillian's file," he explained. But I had read it through twice in the waiting room. The message—almost the exact wording—had seared deeply into my consciousness. A few days later, realizing that the still-vivid details would doubtless fade over time, I reproduced that letter from my memory exactly as it appears here.

Words fail to convey the impact and the devastation of that moment. Knowing my father's life and character, I knew with absolute certainty that those horrendous allegations were not true. I knew that letter contained the most outrageous fabrications ever recorded.

In spite of that fact, huge shock waves of doubt began to inundate my mind, eroding my confidence in myself, my father and my past. I began to question my ability to know anything for certain.

Up to that point in time I had no reason to doubt my sister's honesty, so I ascribed to Lillian equal veracity with my father. For this reason, I was at a loss to explain where these bizarre accusations had come from. I knew they could not have happened as she described them. Yet how could she describe them if they never happened? Could she sincerely believe they had happened if they were not real? Surely she would not make accusations she did not know were true!

I could make no sense of any of it. In total shock, I could not believe this was happening to me. I feared the result of it all could not help but tear the fabric of our family, producing a rend beyond repair.

By now, shock had given way to sheer horror. I realized the drama I had anticipated had turned into a sickening but very real soap opera with a story-line that would devastate my entire family. At any moment that office door would swing open and I would be catapulted onto center stage, still without a script, but now fully aware of the disgusting content of the plot. The way I played my role would have an irrevocable impact on the future of everyone dear to me.

Reason dictated I must settle on a game plan. I dared not allow knee-jerk reaction to prescribe my response. Desperately I begged the Lord for wisdom I did not possess, that I might deal with an alien world which had suddenly engulfed me.

Somehow I knew that when I entered that office there must not be any discernable negative response emanating from my person. Lillian had opened a window that exposed to me what was going on inside of her. If she detected that I had rejected her revelation, she would interpret that to mean I had rejected her, and she would slam the window shut, perhaps never to open it again.

Yet how could I do anything *but* reject these hideous untruths? Repulsion and negation oozed from every pore, screamed from every cell. Every fiber in my body wanted to fight for the honor of my defamed father. I had no desire to lend credence to this garbage by appearing to accept it as fact!

But what of my sister? What could have precipitated her indictment? Dare I risk pushing her back into her reclusion without giving her a fair hearing? Had I the right to judge her before I listened to her, however repulsive and preposterous her story might sound?

On the other hand, how could I insult my gentle father by considering her claim that he was guilty of such crimes against his own daughter?

I detested the fact that I was forced to question the integrity of two people I loved. I revolted at the sure knowledge that one had been flawed at the hand of the other. For if Dad was indeed innocent of Lillian's charges, then she herself emerged as the villain, ruthlessly destroying the character and name of him who gave her life.

How could this allegation of the worst of all debauchery have crept into the inner-sanctum of a God-fearing home? Where was the blessing God had promised to a thousand generations of them that serve Him? Had I not just witnessed the invasion of total degradation somewhere between the first and second generation?

Without a doubt, Dr. French played a significant role in all of this. Waiting outside his office door, I realized I was disadvantaged by meeting with him in his bailiwick. Yet at no time in my life would I again be handed the opportunity to view the world through his and Lillian's eyes. If ever I were to understand my sister, I must embrace this moment to hear her out, distortions and all. It appeared that for the present I must accept her story.

But how could I accept the totally unacceptable? How could I believe what I could not believe? Knowing that grass is green, could I with integrity decide to believe it was red? Never before had the difference between the true and the false seemed so clear, while the choice between right and wrong remained so obscure.

Had I been staring at the contents of Lillian's message for two minutes? Ten? Even twenty? Time did not exist in this alien environment.

I had not yet communicated with Ginny, who was still with me in the waiting room, presumably reading her book. I wondered, how much of this does she know? She gives unwavering support to Lillian. Does she know what is in this note? Does she *believe* what it says?

What about Anna? She also defends Lillian and her doctor. Does she know what Lillian is saying? Does Anna believe it? Worse yet, do they expect *me* to believe it?

Is all the world crazy? Am I crazy?

Hurry, Donna! The door threatens to open any moment! What are you going to do? What will you say?

How I wished it were the door in the TV mystery! How I hoped someone would change the channel!

To stave off panic, I carried on a silent conversation—partly with God, partly with my father and partly with myself.

"Forgive me, Lord, if what I am about to do is wrong. Forgive me, Daddy, if my actions appear to betray you. You are everything that is clean and upright and good. Nobody's lies could change who you are. You would want me to give her a chance, wouldn't you? Forgive me, my Daddy!"

But for the time being, many miles away, Daddy was safe with Mother and Esther Ruth. Right now I must deal with Lillian and this present crisis. I must get inside her head to see what she sees and think what she thinks. I must abandon everything I know, everything I am, to become an empty receptacle, ready to receive the "truth" she and Dr. French are poised to give me. I must abandon my brain in this waiting room. Hopefully, I can retrieve it when I leave!

It was easy enough to decide to spy out the enemy camp, but could I pull it off? Could I shed my true self to become one with them? An old adage advises, "Don't judge a man until you have walked a mile in his shoes." Could I walk in Lillian's and Dr. French's ill-fitting shoes without falling on my face?

Doubts still plagued my mind. Perhaps rather than using reason and logic, I was merely rationalizing. Maybe the best course of action would be to follow my basic instincts and storm in there, yelling, "You are a couple of filthy lying snakes! How dare you accuse my Daddy of such crimes! You are crazy! Really crazy!"

But were they crazy? Could I be the one who is crazy?

The door to Dr. French's office opened. My moment of truth had arrived.

Truth? But what is truth? Hadn't I had just chosen to believe a lie in order to discover truth?

Am I crazy? Are they crazy? Is everybody crazy?

Don't I know any other word besides "crazy?"

CHAPTER TWO

"I Wish You Had Known *My* Daddy"

That Lillian struggled with some sort of problem which caused her to alienate herself from most of her family had been evident for a number of years.

Neither I, nor anyone I knew, had a clue to the nature or origin of Lillian's difficulty. Lillian was my next-in-age sister, two years younger than I. In our family, we girls were generally paired in a biologically-induced buddy system. Lillian and I slept in the same room, often sharing the same bed. We played together and had some of the same friends. Often we received identical Christmas presents, as in the year we each found a baby doll under the tree. Another time, toddler-sized dolls arrived in red and blue velveteen outfits. A year or so later boy dolls completed our "families."

One memorable holiday each of us received a doll carriage, something only children from rich families dared hope for! Yet another Christmas we became joint owners of a doll house, complete with furniture and residents.

That same Christmas our older brother Peter unwrapped a wonderful electric train that puffed real smoke! Lillian and I were delighted to have the train stop beside our doll house and blow its whistle, the signal for an occupant to either board or alight. We were annoyed, however, when he expected passengers *every* time around the track. Didn't he realize our dolls had other things to do besides ride his train?

We were typical kids doing what typical kids do. When Lillian and I were in grade school, I remember when she and Peter argued about Daddy's looks. Five years her senior, Peter was displaying his superior sophistication by informing us that Daddy actually was "ugly."

Our father bore a remarkable resemblance to the pre-whiskered photographs of Abe Lincoln. The likeness was so pronounced that at the age of two, our youngest brother Terry Lee held an envelope bearing a Lincoln stamp and squealed with delight, "Daddy, Daddy!"

Often reminded that he was a Lincoln look-alike, Dad loved to respond by telling of a time Lincoln was traveling alone in his buggy. As another buggy approached from the opposite direction, an astounded Abe watched as, instead of passing on by, the driver pulled alongside and sighted his rifle on him.

Looking down the barrel, Abe's assailant explained, "I always said if I ever met a man uglier than me, I would shoot him."

Without flinching, Lincoln retorted, "If I'm uglier than you, go ahead and shoot."

Perhaps hearing his father tell that story had emboldened Peter to make his declaration. In any event, I am sure Peter was baiting his two younger sisters. Lillian rose grandly to the occasion with proper outrage and genuine tears. "Daddy is *not* ugly! Daddy is *beautiful!*"

Scandalized by their inane argument, I objected, "Daddy is neither ugly nor beautiful. He is Daddy and he looks exactly as Daddy should look." It seemed irreverent to me to reduce him to beauty-contestant status! But Lillian remained both adamant and vocal in her spontaneous defense of her beloved Daddy. A response not to be wondered at—unless, of course, she were not long removed from exploitation by that "beautiful Daddy!"

I saw no change in Lillian while we were living at home. Only after we were both on our own, separated by many miles, did I begin to hear that she felt something other than warmth and acceptance for and from her family. Though Lillian insists that from her earliest years she exhibited the behavior of a mistreated child, I have found no one who knew her then who corroborates that story.

To the contrary, I have questioned various persons who were our mutual friends in those early years. Without exception they verify that they knew Lillian as a happy, well-adjusted girl and teenager who evidenced none of the emotional or behavioral problems she insists she displayed.

This discrepancy in the content of our shared memories had long posed a mystery to me. Before I was aware of the full extent of Lillian's accusations, I knew she struggled with resentments toward her family, particularly her parents.

While I was grieving for Lillian and the death of her childhood, at that same time and miles away, she was suffering a kind of "postpartum depression" due to the birth of her pseudo-childhood. With Dr. French acting as midwife, a long and difficult "labor" had produced their phantom brainchild—long-buried memories of sexual abuse by her father. Now Lillian clutched to her bosom this hideous caricature of her scorned childhood—a greedy parasite that sucked the life from her in its frenzy to sustain and perpetuate itself.

Most of Lillian's brothers and sisters lived too far away to make personal assessments, but we received word from those living close to her that with Dr. French's able assistance, Lillian was making progress toward becoming well. We had no idea the distortions that were being created to induce her progress.

With the welcome news that Lillian was improving, and wanting to assist Lillian regain authentic memories of her home and family, I wrote for her a "memory" of events that we had shared.

Skeletons Without Bones

But even as I wrote, I recognized it to be an exercise in futility, for Dr. French had cautioned us to speak of only surface matters with her. He warned that anything else could trigger a regression, perhaps including an attempt at suicide.

So, with little hope that the message would ever reach its intended audience, I wrote:

I WISH YOU HAD KNOWN **MY** DADDY

To my sister, my very first roommate:

I write this letter to—I don't know who,
For mystery of mysteries, I don't know You.
You—with many faces—some old, some new;
Emerging, withdrawing; now false, now true.
Now we are strangers all the way through
So I don't know who this letter is to.

What I say doesn't matter, I now realize;
So the worth of this letter is naught, I surmise.
Written for you, it will not reach your eyes,
For you can't be exposed to what my memories comprise.
To the rest of the family they contain no surprise.
I can tell "who" and "where" but can answer no "why's."

Whoever you are, Fragile Flower near bloom,
'Tis an awesome task I'm about to assume.
Since we were birthed from the very same womb
Only two years apart, and shared bed and room,
A common childhood we could expect to presume.
Yet my memories bring joy; yours exude gloom.

So I write you a letter you may never read,
But I write it anyway, for I feel the need
To introduce my Daddy. I pray I succeed
In showing him different, quite different indeed,

From the man you have clearly and fiercely decreed
Was an unworthy father who made your heart bleed.

I will abandon the role of poet that I might express my thoughts without restricting them to verse.

For a number of years now I have heard of your family, glimpsing it through your words. I have listened and tried to grasp, to feel, to experience.

But I confess—I cannot understand! Why are you saying these awful things? Why would you make up such hideous lies? If you did not make them up, where did they come from? How can you ever believe such things?[1]

But it is so strange. When you speak, I am told not to contradict you. You must be allowed to express what you know and feel and remember. I am told your memories are real.

Yet when I speak, I am contradicted. I am not allowed to express what I know and feel and remember. My memories are given no validity. Rather, I am accused of being defensive or being in denial or being a Pollyanna! Why am I not attributed the same credibility as you, especially since a large number of brothers and sisters confirm what I say? Are hurting memories the only valid ones? Are good memories always suspect in the Enlightened World of Therapy?

I am not allowed to argue with you. You are You, and your therapist insists that what you claim happened to you, did indeed happen to you! The family you experienced was your family.

But, is it not equally true that "I am I," and my family is my family, every bit as real as yours? And **my** family needs to be introduced, acknowledged, and understood. My family may not have been perfect, but never was it abusive, uncaring or unfeeling. Never was anyone guilty of looking the other way, enabling one family member to victimize another unchallenged or unrestrained.

My very earliest memories of personalities are staged in Baldwinsville. There I remember Dad as the one who crawled under the old shaggy fur coat and became Big Brown Bear—growling and approaching on hands and knees while we thrilled in delightful fright, suspense and horror; knowing it was Daddy, but knowing too it was a Big Brown Bear. We would run and scream, scrambling over each other as we climbed onto the sofa in the semi-darkened room. At last the huge animal reared up, forelegs raised, and the Brown Coat Bear would fall to the floor, now just a brown coat, and Daddy emerged to our relief and delight. The lights came back on, the laughter rang out, and we would squeal, "Do it again, Daddy! Be a Bear again! Please, Daddy."

Now I wonder, Little Fragile Flower, did you laugh and shout and thrill? Or did you only scream and fear, unable to distinguish who was Dad and who was Bear?

I remember Dad as the one who made us a sled—a big brightly-painted bobsled—down in our basement. It was yellow with a big star in the center, its different colored points spreading out in all directions. No one else in our town had such a sled!

On cold snowy evenings we bundled up and pulled our sled the few blocks up the hill near the grade school. There we all piled on the sled four or five deep and down the hill we would fly with Dad at the controls, faster and faster, down several blocks of pure cold fun. Then Dad pulled the sled back uphill as we trudged along, only to pile on and fly down again.

How could it have been otherwise for you? Was the trip too fast, the ride too long, the snowbanks too deep, the thrill too much? Or were you too young to go along, so you stayed at home with Mom, feeling left out and alone while we had all the fun? Perhaps you can't even remember these things, but they must have happened somehow to you, too.

I remember Daddy as devout disciple, spending much time in Bible study and prayer; as faithful employee, catching the early morning bus for work with such regularity that, if Dad was not waiting at the bus stop on a weekday morning, the driver would honk and wait for some signal before he would leave without him.

I remember Daddy bringing home our Bill Ding Blocks[2] and stacking them with us. I later bought an identical set of blocks, ostensibly for my boys. But they were in fact for me—a cherished piece of my childhood. I recall Daddy and Sam Tillotson taking us swimming at Mud Lake in Sammy's old car, for we had none.

We all treasure the times Daddy told us his stories and recited his poems. Warm, fun times of *The Cat, the Dog and the Rooster*[3]; and *Saint Peter Stood Guard at the Golden Gate*[4]; and the one about the old bachelor who went courting[5]. I remember sitting on his knees, thinking how bony they felt, but knowing it was the best place in the world to be!

I remember him reading to the two of us with you on his lap and with me snuggled close to him to see the pictures. I remember the sound and look of his big rough hands as he smoothed each page with a near caress; how his fingers moved to ready the next page to be turned.

Skeletons Without Bones

I remember him calling us pet names. You were Lully Mae; I was Donnie Shay.

Sometimes on payday Daddy brought home new clothes for us. Frequently they reflected his preference for plaids. Your dresses were often blue "to match your eyes," he said. Mine would be pink or red.

I remember Dad as preacher and pastor. When I hear certain passages of Scripture read aloud from the King James Version of the Bible, I still hear them in Daddy's voice and with the cadence of his intonations.

I never walked a chalk line for Daddy or Mother. If a chalk line existed, I never knew it. I didn't feel undue pressure to achieve in school. Rather, I felt that I was expected to get good grades because I was capable of it. No one complained that I had B's sprinkled with an honorable number of A's.

I certainly didn't care to assume the responsibility of a straight A average and I couldn't understand your preoccupation with outstanding scholastic achievement. It appeared to me to be a liability rather than an asset. I can never remember anyone in any way making me feel I could have or should have done better. When I took a report card to Dad for his signature, he would say, "That's fine, Donna, that's fine." And I was content—approved and accepted.

To me, one of Dad's outstanding traits was his obvious and inexplicable pride in each of his children. Even now I can see his expression when we achieved something special, or when someone chanced to make an approving remark about one of us.

I cannot comprehend your feeling of being unloved. To the contrary, I sometimes was embarrassed at Mom and Dad's pride in us. I feared we appeared rather plain and dull to other people. I hoped no one pitied Daddy because his beautiful daughters weren't beautiful at all and his wonderful sons were quite ordinary. But this parental pride and approval was something warm and comfortable to bask in, even if it was a bit unwarranted.

My own place in the sun was winning Dad's reluctant but amused grin. I wasn't cute and smart like Lillian; the only son (in those early years) like Peter; intelligent and literary like Ginny; sweet and loving like Louise; practical and wise like Anna, Daddy's first-born. Neither was I absolutely shockingly unclassifiable like Millie. But I decided I could hold my own in a match of wits, so I sought to capitalize on that. I told myself—without fear of contradiction—that whereas my humor was not so flamboyant and slapstick as Millie's, neither was it as crude and untamed. I concluded mine contained a little more class! Dad's amused grin was my ample reward, even as he sometimes meted out a reprimand or some other form of rebuke. But it was worth it! Dad couldn't quite hide the fact that he appreciated a well-placed remark!

As I grew older, I wasn't afraid to challenge Dad or to disagree with him. Neither was it necessary to rebel. Once in Deanton I ran down the stairs and, jumping the last three or four steps, I landed directly in front of Daddy. Noting my flushed face, he asked as he rubbed my cheek, "Is that nature or drug-store?" Innocent of the implied misdemeanor—make-up was a no-no in those days—and feeling cocky at his unwitting compliment, I looked him in the eye and said, "You mean you can't even **tell?!**" He didn't reply, but we both knew I had scored the point.

Dad was strict and conservative himself, but he never forced it on us kids once he judged us old enough to make our own decisions. I felt no pressure to be anyone but myself, and myself was acceptable.

One more thing still vivid in my mind was Dad's excitement when one of the older girls came home for a visit. He could scarcely wait for the arrival and his comment was always, "She's lookin' good, isn't she?" Of course, Dad thought we looked good with stringy hair, hand-me-down clothes and runny noses!

But there always followed the inevitable sad ending, the day the "visitor" must leave again. I can still see Dad standing on the porch plucking at his chin whiskers, staring off into space, feeling blue because one of his children had just left for college or home. And I would hurt for him, knowing we were loved and cherished—each and every one.

To illustrate, one Christmas about thirty years ago we kids were excited about the presents under the tree, as usual, and Mother kept restraining us as we poked, pinched, speculated and counted. But Dad was the most excited "kid" of all that year, keeping track of one particular gift he had singled out from among the rest. He asked Mom if he could open the thin, rectangular package early, "Since I know what it is anyway." Mother said, "No, you have to wait like everyone else!"

That was what Mom thought! In the midst of supper preparations that Christmas Eve, someone chanced into the almost-deserted front room, and furtively motioned us all to come—"Shhh!" We tiptoed to the doorway. There was Daddy, flat on his stomach on the floor, his head surrounded by the low branches of our Christmas tree. With discarded wrapping paper beside him as indisputable evidence of his crime, he gazed lovingly at the likenesses of his first little grandchildren—golden-haired Nancy and raven-haired Rosie—whom, if I am not mistaken, he had never actually seen. Mother scolded, we children laughed and teased, but Daddy just grinned his grin, looking as guilty as sin. Without repentance or remorse, he held up his booty as if he were displaying a hard-won trophy.

This, then, is **my** Daddy—human, fun, real, and good. I witness before heaven and earth, Lillian, that this was your Daddy, too.

I am sorry you fail to remember him as he was and that you refuse to claim the "genuine article" as your father, too. For some reason perhaps known only to yourself, you have sold both your birthright and your blessing for a mess of psychological pottage.

I grieve for you and your irreplaceable loss. I also grieve for Daddy. In these, his final years as Alzheimer's disease takes its toll, he must feel his irreplaceable loss, too.

Isn't it a mystery—in our teeming, boisterous household—you never knew my Daddy. And I never caught a glimpse of yours.[6]

CHAPTER THREE

In the Viper's Den

As Dr. French came through his office door into the waiting room, I waived aside his caution that I be gentle with Lillian.

What did the man take me for, a total fool? Of course I would be gentle with her. I considered her as much his victim as was Daddy, although in her case it was volitional. I was outraged because of Lillian's accusations against our father. Later my outrage would intensify as she would choose to remain under Dr. French's tutelage in spite of national headlines making public his use of "sex therapy" with his female clients.

Yet with my anger co-existed concern. She was my sister. I loved her and admired many things about her. I desired for her the liberation of knowing the truth—truth about her past, her parents and herself. Dr. French had nothing to fear. I would be gentle with her.

He motioned me to the door and I entered the viper's den. My sister cowered in the corner of a large overstuffed chair as I approached her and knelt on one knee in front of her. The first words out of her mouth questioned, "Donna, do you believe me?"

Ah, there it was. With no time to hedge or hesitate, I ventured, "I certainly don't think you could have thought that up by yourself." She looked relieved, missing my oblique reference to the role of her psychologist. And I had not lied. So far, so good!

Her next question was, "How do you feel?"

I surprised myself by responding, "I feel as if I would like to put my arms around you and hold you."

Since she did not visibly respond to that remark and since I had been previously warned by Dr. French not to physically touch her, I continued to kneel in front of her, resting my elbow on the arm of the great chair. This provided a sense of intimacy without touching.

Her questions kept coming. "How do you feel about Daddy now?"

I looked her straight in the eye and said, "I feel very, very sorry for him." Again I had told the absolute truth, leaving her to her own interpretation. I believe the Lord helped me maintain communication without falsehoods and without confrontation.

Some have criticized me, saying I was false with Lillian at that moment. I understand their position; they can never understand mine. I have relived that scene a hundred times over. Even with the clarity of hindsight, were I given a chance to re-play my part in that drama, I cannot imagine how I would do it differently. Except this time I would put my arms around my sister and cry with her—and let French go hang.

I'm not sure what else we said as I remained kneeling before her chair. Sisters who had not communicated at a deep level for as many as twenty years, we had to feel our way along with caution.

We could not have come from more divergent paths. Immersed in the concepts of Janov's book *The Primal Scream*[1] and similar material, and guided by Dr. French, Lillian had for a number of years scavenged through the gutters of "intensive therapy." The purpose of this unconventional method of therapy seemed to include locating and identifying specimens of raw family sewage extracted from ancient burial sites deep within Lillian's psyche. These specimens were subsequently scrutinized, codified and interpreted by Dr. French, who then exhibited them to Lillian as relics of her past, positive proof of her early victimization.

Those same years my husband and I had traveled in an itinerant ministry, preaching and singing in churches and crusades across the United States. As opportunity allowed, we visited relatives and close friends along the way. We spent hours reminiscing over days gone by, looking at photographs and catching up on news of common friends and acquaintances. We laughed at odd family traits, marveled at common foibles and compared uncommon characteristics. We reviewed our sorrows, shared our losses and mourned our broken relationships. Through it all, we found only typical and generally wholesome stuff. We stumbled upon no sordid pasts; we uncovered no buried traumas. No closeted skeletal remains leered at us as together we opened long-closed doors of our past.

Recognizing more and more the priceless heritage my parents had provided for their offspring through care and prayer, I knew nothing of the sewer of bogus memories in which Lillian was nearly drowning.

Those divergent paths Lillian and I had traveled unexpectantly converged in Dr. French's office, where I sought to establish myself as an unresisting student of the "superior knowledge" my sister and her therapist thrust upon me.

Lillian's journey back into her buried memories had been presided over by a much-experienced tour guide in the person of Dr. French. I asked Dr. French if from the beginning of Lillian's therapy, he had known she had been molested by her father. He assured me that, as is true with all professional counselors, he knew nothing except what the client disclosed to him.

With that disclaimer on the table, I tried a different approach, appealing directly to his ego. "But certainly, Dr. French, you could not have been taken by surprise? With your experience and expertise, you must have suspected she had been abused long before she actually remembered it."

And he bit. He confessed that right away he had presumed her father had molested her when she was very young.

That admission confirmed to me my suspicions that he had purposefully and relentlessly steered my sister through the maze of his tainted therapy toward a predetermined destination—incest.

Thus, in the tribunal of the doctor's mind, my father had been declared guilty long before my sister had leveled a charge. So much for his pretention to know nothing except what he learned from the client!

Back when I first learned of my sister's accusations, the term "recovered repressed memories" had yet to be coined. Now more than a decade later, numerous articles and books have been and continue to be published, showing agreement with my early conclusions that so-called recovered memories would more accurately be designated "therapy-implanted memories."[2]

In an effort to glean more tidbits from Dr. French's mind, I asked, "Why would my father single out Lillian, daughter number six, to be his only victim?"

Dr. French explained, "Differences in children's personalities affect how they interact with adults and influence how adults respond to them." My sister Ginny, for instance, had filled the role of "placator," as she performed in all the ways she felt were expected of her. He cited Ginny's early literary interests as attempts to gain the notice of a disinterested father.

My thoughts time-warped back to those quiet evenings in Baldwinsville, New York, when we younger children played on the floor while Daddy and Ginny sat on the sofa and read aloud together Sir Walter Scott's *Lady of the Lake*. A perfectly happy memory had just been twisted to conform to Dr. French's fantasy of our "dysfunctional family."

Dr. French further confided that Ginny's problems for which he had counseled her a dozen or so years stemmed from our father's neglect to hold and cuddle her as a baby.

It amazed me that this remarkable man could literally see into the past. How could he conclude Daddy never held Ginny? He wasn't there! Studies reveal that we retain no memories during our first six months,[3] so Ginny could not be the source of that knowledge. Dr. French had never questioned anyone, either in our family or out, who could have had that knowledge. Yet unencumbered by facts or conscience, he confidently enlightened me with "truth" he could not possibly substantiate.

In the Viper's Den

Early in Mother's first pregnancy her appendix ruptured. In spite of an emergency appendectomy, she succeeded in carrying the baby to full term.

The infant, named Virginia, cried with colic her entire first six weeks. Since Mother was not immediately able to care for a newborn and two small step-daughters, Daddy assumed most of Ginny's care, alternating between rocking her and walking the floor with her. Thus, in the real world, the father who in Dr. French's diagnosis had never held his infant daughter had in fact held her almost constantly for six solid weeks!

Now that I knew Dr. French's version of Ginny's history, I could scarcely wait to hear his rendition of mine. Not surprisingly, the revered doctor had a label for me also. He described me as a "Pollyanna," with characteristics like my mother. He said I had succeeded in keeping my lecherous father at bay by exhibiting a happy-go-lucky, "everything is fine even when it isn't" type of disposition.

Once again, the man astounded me! On the occasions we had met, he had either ignored me or fleetingly treated me with disdain. Now I discovered he not only knew what I was like, but he knew in what ways I was like my mother!

To top it all, Lillian informed me that Daddy was only attracted to "cute little girls." It didn't take a Mensa mentality to figure out that of Daddy's seven daughters, she alone qualified! To bolster her premise, she reminded me of Daddy's fondness for Jeanette.

I wondered what they would do if I were to become sick all over that office.

When we lived in Upstate New York, my parents were approved to provide foster home care. Often, the state called to urge Mother to accept one more child in need of a stable, loving environment. This happened in spite of the fact that New York State was bending its own rule which limited the number of children that could be placed in any given home.

Four of the twelve children my parents raised to adulthood were foster children in need of long-term care. Eventually my folks

Skeletons Without Bones

became their legal guardians, but they belonged to us long before the court decreed it.

Other children came to us on a short-term basis, expected to soon return to their parents. Still others we kept as they were prepared for adoption. The state always informed us of the status of each child so we would not become unduly attached to one we could not expect to keep.

A newborn named Jeanette was placed with us while legalities were being completed for her adoption. Her stay stretched to two and one-half years and we watched her grow into a petite "Dresden doll" with dark curls that bounced as she walked. Partly because she was irresistible both in appearance and in disposition, and partly because we knew she could be taken from us at any time, Jeanette became everybody's pet. In spite of New York's precautions, we all became unduly attached. Daddy was no exception. Often he carried her on his shoulders from where she reigned, our undisputed little queen.

When they took her from us, we were inconsolable. For Mother it proved to be more difficult than losing her to death. Public gatherings and shopping trips became torturous exercises of searching the crowds for the little girl we had loved and lost.

Scavenging through Lillian's past in search of filth, Dr. French had leaped upon Daddy's attachment for Jeanette, labeling it "illicit." Dr. French concluded the Welfare Department had removed her from our home for her own personal safety. I wondered if any legitimate affection could survive passage through Dr. French's sewage-sodden mind.

In real life, as Jeanette approached her third birthday, and with her adoption still on hold, her birth mother's religious preference needed to be obliged. Jeanette was transferred from our Protestant home to a Catholic home. It was as simple as that.

If I had been quick enough to ask Dr. French why the welfare took Jeanette from us and let us have Marie, would he have said that Marie, like the rest of us girls, simply failed the cute test?

When I heard French's explanation of Jeanette's departure from our home, my incredulity must have been evident. What else could

In the Viper's Den

have prompted Dr. French to blurt out, "Your father had that house full of girls—what the h— was he *supposed* to do?"

WHAT??!! I could not believe my ears! The man who had helped reduce my sister to a zombie by identifying my father as her molester now suggested to me that Daddy had done the only thing that could be expected of any red-blooded male faced with the same tantalizing opportunity!

"What was he *supposed* to do?", Dr. French asked. The obvious answer is, he was supposed to love and protect them; teach and nurture them; clothe, house, and feed them; and bring them up in the nurture and admonition of the Lord. An awesome responsibility—but that is exactly what he did do for all seven of his little girls and his five little boys.

That's what he was supposed to do and he did it consistently, selflessly and willingly, with no exceptions and no glitches—just as countless other decent, loving fathers have done since the beginning of time.

Dr. French also had daughters. Using his own terminology and his own suppositions, one feels compelled to ask, "What the h— did *YOU* do, Dr. French?"

Not many years after we lost Jeanette, Mother received the astounding news that at forty-nine years of age, she was pregnant! When the fullness of time had come, Terry Lee made his dramatic appearance into our home. At age fifty-seven, once again Daddy became the doting father and soon Terry, his constant companion, assumed Jeanette's vacated throne atop Daddy's shoulders.

I wonder, will we someday hear from Lillian via Dr. French that Dad also had an inappropriate attachment for "cute little boys"?

They had not yet finished with their rewriting of our history. One memory preeminent in the minds of all Dad's children is that of waking early in the morning and hearing the sounds of our Daddy in prayer. He would be on his knees and on cold mornings he knelt over a hot air register.

The sounds were not loud. We heard muffled sighs and whispered words, and perhaps a muted groan. Unable to make out the actual words of his prayer, we children were sure he talked to his heavenly Father about each one of us. We knew that between the two of them, none of our deeds escaped full notice and evaluation in the ramparts of heaven. This knowledge often prompted Daddy's offspring to make mid-course corrections as we journeyed through childhood.

Again I sickened as Dr. French explained that Dad's early morning trysts occurred as he was repeatedly tortured out of his sleep by a conscience still convulsing from unconfessed violations of his daughter.

Had Dr. French possessed integrity enough to ask, he would have learned that Daddy's early morning prayer vigils were well established long before the birth of this one "cute little girl."

Neither was Mother to escape their negation. In accusatory tones Lillian presented proof that Mother didn't love her by declaring, "Donna, the last time Mother visited me, *she didn't even touch me!*"

My eyes shifted to Dr. French. Hampered neither by conscience nor integrity, his impassive stare never hinted that he intended to make his own confession. Aghast, I ventured one for him.

"Of course Mother never touched you! When I knelt in front of you, I never touched you either! Do you not know your great counselor has placed an impenetrable wall around you? In this very office he *forbade* Mother to touch you."

Mother and I had accompanied Ginny on one of her weekly appointments. Dr. French had used his typical intimidating tactics to bring my mother under his control. When she had objected, "She is my daughter. Can't I touch her if I want to?," he replied with the authority of the law of the Medes and Persians. "Yes, you can," he said. "But if you love her, you won't!"

It galled me to see him handle members of my family much as a master chessman moves his pawns to his own advantage. Yet, pointing out to Lillian a clear example of his duplicity had no effect on her. No wonder Dr. French didn't bother to defend himself to her. He knew he didn't need to.

In the Viper's Den

When I asked, "Dr. French, was my mother aware of my father's abuse?", in his best condescension he suggested, "Maybe you should ask *her* that question."

I reminded him, "Since it is not now possible for me to question my mother, would you tell me your opinion as to whether she knew?"

He obliged me by saying, "Your Mother could not help but know what was going on. But possessing no courage and little concern, she turned her head rather than cause ripples. *But surely she knew!*"

Furthermore, he informed me that other people knew also. Had it never occurred to me there might be a reason Daddy had found it necessary to move from one church to another rather than stay in one place during the years of his ministry?

Sometimes Dr. French's questions were too moronic to warrant a response. No, I had never been suspicious of the reasons we moved. The wonder is that Dr. French posed the inane question. It was so much a custom of that era for pastors to move every few years that annual conferences, church congregations and pastoral families all factored into their calendars and lives the possibility of a move.

Conversations around a typical parsonage were punctuated with statements such as, "If we are still here next year," and, "I hope we don't move before I graduate," and, "Maybe our next parsonage will have two bathrooms."

Church members were no less acclimated. "We had hoped the hot water tank in the parsonage would hold up until the next pastoral change;" or, "Doesn't the pastor sing (play or teach) well? I don't know what we'll do when they leave." Or even, "It's been awhile since we've had children in the parsonage. I hope our next pastor has kids."

The conference or district officials were acutely aware of frequent pastoral changes which often occurred at conference time. Early spring they began compiling two significant lists: one list of pastors who needed new pastoral assignments that year and another list of churches that needed new pastors. The goal was to

Skeletons Without Bones

match available churches with available pastors and come out even—with everyone reasonably satisfied with the arrangements.

One might excuse Dr. French's ignorance of church practice if he had not previously been an ordained Methodist minister back East. I pose a counter question concerning Dr. French. Why, as a young pastor, did he surrender his ministerial credentials, change careers, and move 3,000 miles from one coast to the other? Perhaps the reason he so easily cast suspicion on others was to keep the searchlight off his own murky past!

Another line of attack used by my father's saboteurs concerned Daddy's writings. Lillian asked, "Donna, have you ever read Daddy's books."

"Of course I have read them."

"What did you *think* of his horrid books?"

Her question took me off guard. I certainly didn't think what her emphasis and inflections insinuated I *should* think.

Dr. French took advantage of my hesitation by telling me that anyone with half a brain could tell those books were written by a sick mind.

Not everyone shared Dr. French's evaluation of Daddy's material or his mind. I don't think Dad ever submitted a manuscript to our denominational magazine but that they published it, and he submitted many. Granted, Daddy didn't write for the man on the street. He was a Biblical scholar and a theologian, evidenced by the inclusion of one of his books on the collateral reading list for theology students at an evangelical seminary.

After I had sampled Dr. French's required reading for his clients, including some items that he had authored, I was confident Dad would have been gratified to know his books had merited the doctor's scathing review.

My father's literary critic had made some astounding discoveries about my father's teaching, also. He asked me if I knew about the "Bride of Christ."

Without a context I did not know how to answer that question. You could not grow up in our home without knowing about the Bride of Christ and just about every other Biblical topic you could mention. But since nothing spoken in that office had yet made sense to me, I didn't expect to be on Dr. French's wave length now.

Again he asked if I knew what "the Bride of Christ" meant. I cautiously asserted I knew what the Bible said about it.

"But did you know your father told Lillian she was never to marry because *she* was to become the Bride of Christ?" Dad, Dr. French declared, thought himself to be some sort of forerunner on the order of John the Baptist and together they—Dad and Lillian—were to prepare the world for Christ's coming!

Furthermore, Dr. French said Lillian had been told by our father that she must commit the entire Bible to memory so that when the last copy of Scripture had been destroyed, it could be reproduced from the depository of Lillian's memory.

Once again the realization overwhelmed me that insanity was the norm and reality was a stranger to the world where Dr. French reigned!

Was it any wonder that Dr. French told me not to divulge to my family what he and Lillian were telling me? Is it any wonder I have never, until this writing, told anyone the whole story of what took place in that office that day? Who would believe such a wild tale? Who could help but question *my* grasp on reality?

My father was respected as a Bible teacher in the denomination by which he had been ordained. Whether he taught a large crowd, a small Bible study, or his own children at home, Dad was always Biblically sound and thoroughly orthodox. Contrary to Dr. French and Lillian, he correctly taught that the Bride of Christ is the complete body of believers—the church universal. He never believed the Bride was a literal woman, certainly not his own daughter!

Dad was so consistent, so totally without deviation in his theology and in the personal living-out of his theology, that as a young child I was always awe-struck when he would recite *Saint Peter at the Gate.*

The poem depicts a man and woman arriving at the gate of heaven. She had been a loyal, albeit obnoxious, church member

Skeletons Without Bones

all her life. In spite of, and perhaps because of, her constant nagging, the husband had not bothered with things religious.

Never at a loss for words, the wife immediately attacked the celestial gate guard with her ever-sharp tongue and her ever-ready opinions. When Saint Peter could interrupt the woman's stream of verbiage, he refused her entrance into heaven, directing her toward the regions below. Without a question, the man turned to follow. If her religious exercises had not sufficed for her, what hope had he to gain admittance?

But Saint Peter detained him with a question. "How long have you been married to that woman?" When the man confessed it had been thirty years, Saint Peter made an instant executive decision and ushered the astonished man through the Pearly Gates with the explanation, "This poor soul has endured all the hell he needs!"

The poem is pure entertainment, in no way intended to withstand theological scrutiny. Still, it always amazed me that my by-the-Book father would recite such a poem, even in jest—let alone that he would take such obvious delight in doing so!

Lest my point be more obscure than obvious, I contend that in our household, our father could not stray from his normally sound, thoroughly orthodox interpretation of anything remotely theological, even in fun, without every one of his children being fully aware of his heresy. How delighted we would have been if we could have once caught our daddy in the tiniest Biblical digression! We would *never* have let it die!

So why, only after years of therapy, did Lillian suddenly recall horrific deviations from Dad's usual impeccable knowledge and application of Scripture?

The answer is simple. Her "memories" were not memories at all. They were fabrications of a therapist eager to ply his trade on a patient willing to accept any explanation that exempted her from taking responsibility for problems in her life. Though I may not have known the term "therapy-induced recovered repressed memories,"[4] I knew Dr. French's influence had left Lillian brainwashed beyond my comprehension.

In the Viper's Den

During the last tirade about the Bride of Christ, Dr. French had been the speaker. Afterward, Lillian added that Dad had instructed her that she should remain single and become a missionary doctor. They explained that, "Dad had fashioned for Lillian a career both holy and celibate, in an attempt to 'save her for himself,' indicative of his continued sexual interest in her. Then, when the proper time came, the two of them would prepare the world for Jesus' coming and Lillian would become the 'Bride of Christ!'"

Someone obviously *had* been messing with Lillian's mind! I knew the culprit had *not* been my father.

Becoming sick all over French's office would have been too kind!

CHAPTER FOUR

Dr. French: Friend or Fraud?

When a loved one becomes so mesmerized by an authority figure that total dependency for guidance and affirmation rests with that authority figure, family members naturally become suspicious and even alarmed. Dr. French had held a controlling interest in Ginny and Lillian's lives for so long, it had become difficult to imagine them without his overshadowing influence.

Dr. French first came into our lives by way of my sister Ginny. Because Ginny's desire to live a Christian life was often sabotaged by her equally strong desire to be free of outside restrictions, the resulting conflict became one of the reasons she sought help through counseling.

Ginny originally had consulted a revered friend and pastor whom she felt would provide counsel from a Christian perspective and with a Biblical base. Convinced that Pastor Don Ensonique was providing the help she sought, Ginny rejoiced in her spiritual and emotional growth. Comparing notes over the phone with her sister Lillian, they together concluded that Lillian also would benefit from Pastor Don's counsel.

A Christmas visit to the Northwest confirmed their original opinion, so in the early 1970's Lillian's husband moved his family several thousand miles to obtain help for his floundering wife. As far as I know, for many of us this was the first inkling we had—sketchy and vague as it was—that Lillian struggled with any sort of difficulty. However, our concern was tempered with the knowledge she would receive help from Ginny's pastor and support from close family members.

Pastor Ensonique found Lillian's condition to be beyond his level of expertise and he recommended she make an appointment with Dr. French. Pastor Ensonique felt Ginny also would benefit from Dr. French's counsel, so both sisters became clients of this highly recommended "Christian psychologist."

Dr. French was born in India to missionary parents toward whom, according to his adherents, he bears more than a little resentment. He received his education in India and Europe. Records show he obtained ministerial credentials and pastored in both Presbyterian and Methodist churches in the northeastern United States.

Although he has touted himself as a Christian psychologist and has produced what he calls an integration of Christianity and psychology, Dr. French's writings reveal the pronounced influence of an Eastern, Hindu-dominated culture.

Some time into their therapy, my sisters began to give glowing reports of this paragon of love, wisdom, understanding and truth. He was able to take perceived triteness and obscurity of Scripture, flood it with the pure light of his psycho-theology, and produce insights that lesser luminaries could scarcely hope to discover.

For instance, Dr. French judged Moses, King David, John the Beloved and even the Apostle Paul as not being psychologically whole, which would explain their inability to say what they meant, or to understand what they said. Dr. French, on the other hand, could define or redefine their terminology and decipher their intent. Better yet, he could psychoanalyze them and explain what better men they could have been had they had access to his superior insight.

Dr. French's own persona was replete with contradictions. A former client observed, "There is no middle ground regarding people's opinion of him. One either adores him or one detests him."

My contacts with him prior to my appointment in his office with Lillian in 1979 bore out the truth of that observation. Among my sisters' acquaintances, I found myself alone in voicing suspicions of him, primarily because many of their friends were also disciples of Dr. French. Their loyalty to him bordered on fanatical and they assigned him no guilt when I described his caustic badgering of me when he had interviewed me. They interpreted my reaction to him as evidence of my prejudice; any flaw resided in my character, not his.

We could not have had more opposite opinions of one person. Whereas my sisters found him loving and gentle, to me he had been brusque and sarcastic. To them he was strong and wise; I considered him an insipid old fool. They saw his extreme patience; I figured dispensing patience at his prices scarcely constituted a virtue.

While they believed he interpreted Scripture with rare insight, I cringed at the way he twisted it to support his own heresies. They tolerated his arrogance with fond amusement; I felt his egotism had been astutely characterized by my son who described Dr. French as an "alpha male."

Lest I appear to consider myself wiser than fact would warrant, let me insert a confession. I too have been fooled, believing in the integrity and genuine Christian morality of persons who later proved to be wolves in sheep's clothing.

That experience of misplaced trust now prompted me to assume the role of an investigative reporter, searching out empirical evidence regarding both Dr. French and my father. As we resumed our itinerary, I asked questions and gathered information along the way. I was convinced that whether Dad was guilty or innocent, the facts would become obvious under scrutiny. I hoped I was prepared to face the consequences if I had misjudged either man.

Dr. French had numerous interesting, if unorthodox, interpretations of Scripture. He explained that Abraham had such deep-seated emotional problems, only God's direct intervention prevented him from murdering his own son. To Dr. French, Abraham may appear unstable and in need of psychological adjustment, but because of Abraham's unflinching obedience, God displayed him as a trophy in his Hall of Fame.[1] Clearly, Dr. French flunked "Interpretation of Scripture 101." When he questioned the truth of a statement made by the Apostle Paul, Ginny reminded him that Paul had said, *"All Scripture is God-breathed."*[2] Dr. French responded, "Yes, but I think God sometimes had a hard time breathing through Paul's lungs."

Dr. French claimed that his blend of psychology and Christianity now formed a bridge over which persons could pass to meet God. Were we to believe that the position Christ had filled throughout history as "the Way" to God had now been taken over by Dr. French?

Once I had asked Lillian, "Does your Christian counselor ever use Scripture in his dealing with you? Does he ever pray with you?"

She replied, "No, he doesn't use the Bible. He told me I don't need to read the Bible anymore." As for prayer, she said, "I can't even discuss such things with you because when I use the word 'prayer,' it has a totally different meaning than you mean by the word."

If Dr. French deemed the reading of the Bible as unnecessary, he felt quite differently about Janov's *Primal Scream*, which was required reading for his clients. I purchased the book, forcing my way through four chapters of muck before putting it aside forever. I couldn't imagine how reading that psychobabble could help anyone get well; it made me sick. Each time I read from it, I felt I was being dragged through an enormous cesspool.

Dr. French advocated and used primal therapy, and *The Primal Scream* was his textbook. Many of his clients were subjected to his own version of "intensive therapy." After reading *Primal Scream* at least once, the patient was secluded in a remote cabin for three to six weeks. No distractions such as radios, telephones, stereos or televisions were permitted. Reading material was limited to assignments given by Dr. French.

Supplies, purchased ahead of time, consisted only of food and writing materials. During confinement the client went nowhere and saw no one except Dr. French. Daily therapy sessions were held either in his office or in the seclusion of the cabin.

The purpose of all this isolation was to "get in touch with one's feelings." With all the sordid testimonials and accompanying interpretations given in *The Primal Scream* freshly implanted in her mind, the client was instructed to explore the possibility of undiscovered incest or molestation in her childhood, all the way back to the time of birth.

The client was instructed to "talk to her parents," and journal her thoughts and feelings, all of which was subsequently dissected and interpreted by the psychologist. Many times the process was enhanced by the use of drugs or hypnosis or both.

Not surprisingly, a remarkable number of persons emerged from these sessions with "recovered memories" of sexual abuse and incest which purportedly had long been buried somewhere deep within.[3]

To question the methods, motives or morals of a psychologist, especially one who calls himself Christian, invites disaster. But even a casual student of brainwashing or mind control techniques would instantly recognize the dangers inherent in the above scenario.

So it was not only Dr. French's theological or Biblical interpretations that caused concern. His psychological concepts and methodology encompassed everything intimated by the phrase "from the sublime to the ridiculous."

One tenet which he espoused assumed all physical ailments derived from psychological roots. Dr. French believes when a person reaches psychological wholeness, physical wholeness results as a natural consequence. While most people accede that the two aspects of a person are intrinsically related and interacting, Dr. French seemed to carry the concept to a fanatical and unrealistic extreme. It interested me to find that the Doctor himself suffered an increasing hearing loss he could not reverse and about which he seemingly was "in denial." Apparently he was incapable of demonstrating the validity of his own dogma.

Many people, including myself, have noticeably improved their health by making changes in their lifestyle and eating habits. Without the use of any psychological hocus-pocus, various physical symptoms of long duration often improve or even completely disappear when we adopt a healthier way of life.

Such disciplines would be far too simplistic for one of Dr. French's persuasion. Besides, if potential clients could improve their physical health and well-being without long years of expensive therapy, it would leave him out of the food chain! It is easy to understand his prejudice.

Dr. French's custom of assigning double meanings to words or phrases in order to diagnose psychological problems appeared to me to be more cutesy than legitimate. For example, taking their cues from Dr. French, it was common practice among my sisters' families to attempt to cure whatever ailed them by psychologically interpreting their physical problems. When they developed colds, they believed it indicated they had recently felt "left out in the cold." If they could identify the occasion and "process it," they claimed they could eliminate the cause of their colds and thereby recover.

Treated or untreated, colds do eventually go away, rendering it impossible to prove or disprove that their psychological voodoo impacted the recovery process. Nevertheless, their confidence remained undimmed.

The possibilities of finding psychological clues to physical problems are endless, limited only by one's acuity at turning a phrase. For instance, if you develop a fever blister, you merely determine when it was you repressed the desire to make a blistering remark to someone, resolve the conflict and you have a fever blister on the mend.

Of course, if you labeled your malady a cold sore rather than a fever blister, you would need to alter the remedy to match the altered terminology.

Dr. French: Friend or Fraud

When I had caught on to the concept, I decided to try my hand at it. Tongue-in-cheek, I told my sister Ginny that now I understood a puzzling phenomenon stemming from our childhood.

In an earlier chapter I spoke of the natural occurrence of a genetically-induced buddy system within our family. Three sets of sisters were paired in that manner. Anna and Louise were the two eldest, followed by Ginny and Millie. Peter slipped in there solo, followed by myself and Lillian to complete the final set of sisters.

Crowding several children into limited numbers of bedrooms compelled each pair of sisters to share a common double bed. By some quirk of fate, one sister in each pair had the disgusting tendency to wet the bed at night. This malady was not looked upon with fondness by the "dry" sister. I suspect it was as unpleasant to the unoffending partner as it was to the perpetrator, but I had no way to check the truth of that statement.

But now, years later, I decided to apply Dr. French's formula to those not-yet-forgotten, scarcely-forgiven soggy scenarios of our youth.

Perhaps good could be salvaged from the memories of my disgrace when in the wee hours, expediency forced me to awaken my blissfully-sleeping sister. I suppose the offending fluid could not be faulted for seeking the path of least resistance, even if it did cross that oft-defined equator that separated the hemispheres of our bed. By nature, and perhaps by cultivation, Lillian had possessed the sweeter disposition of the two of us, but that fact was not easily discerned in dimly-lit, pre-dawn hours.

No doubt the self-righteousness and disdain that oozed from her person were as impossible to hold in check as was the offending fluid originating with my person!

At any rate, self-esteem is only a therapist's pipe-dream when at two in the morning you are stripping yourself and your bed of dripping bed clothes. You desperately hope that this event has not already occurred tonight in too many of the other bedrooms in the house. Scarcity of clean linen is too horrible a fate to contemplate at that hour.

Since dry sisters become volatile if kept vertical longer than three nocturnal minutes, you must rush from one bed corner to another, pulling and tucking sheets and blankets at top speed while the offended sister shivers both visibly and audibly. You learn early on that to solicit her help only adds insult to injury. Besides, you want her to remain in her zombie-like near-sleep mode, for zombies seldom transfer data from short-term to long-term memory banks in the middle of the night, which makes for more amiable mornings-after.

Since Ginny in the role of offended zombie and Millie as bed-changer had endured similar midnight rendezvous, I thought I was outrageously funny as I theorized on the significance of those occasions.

I explained to Ginny that the malady known as bed-wetting was no malady at all. It was a spontaneous cleansing of the psyche which, while *irritating* to bed partners, was *irrigating* to the perpetrators. While Ginny and Lillian had dammed up their problems inside to their future detriment, Millie and I had blissfully eliminated all our hang-ups by night. The next day it was simply a matter of adding soap and water and our troubles were washed away, never to bother us again. Hence, in our adult years, Millie and I had not found it necessary to pay a therapist top dollar to expose and eradicate our neuroses, for they had been flushed out years before.

Ginny's response to my hilarity caught me off guard. Rather than join my laughter, she said Dr. French would likely agree that had been the case! The next time I accompanied Ginny to Dr. French's office, I told him of my fanciful diagnosis of our bed-wetting experience. As Ginny had predicted, he nodded wisely and said I was right—that is exactly what had happened!

I was embarrassed for him that for such wisdom he had spent years in college! I could see I had missed my calling!

Dr. French enjoyed notoriety beyond his immediate locale. He annually conducted six-week seminars in an evangelical theological seminary in southern California. He helped establish a Graduate School of Psychology on campus and the building erected to house the department proudly bore his name. A well-known corporation from the Northwest had donated the money for the building, stipulating how the structure should be christened. It was no coincidence that the donor company's name was also the last name of a long-term colleague of Dr. French.

Dr. French's influence over his clients was not confined to his office and the cabins used for intensive therapy. Semi-annual retreats were held in various conference centers. For many of his patients, to miss summer conference or winter retreat was tantamount to deep deprivation. Neither these conferences nor the intensive therapy came cheap, but Dr. French further endeared himself to his followers by offering scholarships to selected worthy adherents, thereby ensuring their gratitude as well as their continued indoctrination.

To even the casual observer, a definite cult-like dimension dominated Dr. French's relationship with his clients. Their devotion was complete, their loyalty fanatical. He became everything to them, so infiltrating their lives that he was more family to them than were their blood relatives.

It is impossible to exaggerate his domination of the entire lives of a large number of his clients. He unblushingly jockeyed for the privilege to give away a bride in lieu of her own natural and living father, creating a schism the woman was unable to heal before her father's death. Regret evidenced by her tears, she testified under oath of the breach that still existed between her and her family caused by Dr. French's intrusiveness.

Dr. French always had access to babies who needed placement in homes. He regularly presented the needs of these infants to clients and arranged for their adoptions by his clients whenever possible.

One set of adoptive parents confessed to us they had been so enamored by their therapist that when the French family was expected for a visit at their farm, the husband would scrub the walls of the horse stalls in the barn in preparation for their coming guests. Noting our amazement, he said with apparent chagrin, "That is what you do if 'God' is coming for a visit!"

Skeletons Without Bones

Dr. French sometimes became provider and financier for his clients, either by extending to them substantial loans or making outright grants of money. They reciprocated by plying him with gifts and demonstrating their undying gratitude.

And how they loved him. They remained his loyal patients for periods of ten, fifteen, twenty years and longer. They were always said to be improving, learning and progressing, but never got well to the point of not needing more therapy.[4] Dr French blatantly claimed that he alone held the key to their complete healing. The longer it took, the more they vouched for his extra-ordinary patience and loving concern.

They never questioned whether decades of therapy might indicate a flaw in the validity of the cure or a glitch in the effectiveness of the therapist. The unusual length of time it required to become well was to them an indication of the depth of their neuroses. Who else would have hung in there with them for such an extended period of time? That he collected a nice hefty fee for each visit seemed not to diminish their gratitude.

Besides, who among them wanted to be so cured they no longer needed their doctor? Not one of them that I ever met or heard about. Dr. French admitted as much to me once when I asked him if Lillian would ever be well. He said, "Lillian is as well as she wants to be." I silently added, "And as well as you want her to be."

I later learned I was not alone in my suspicions of Dr. French's character and methodology. In order to verify that he indeed had good credentials, in the early 1980's my husband and I called the office responsible for the licensing of professionals in Washington State. By merely stating that we had relatives under Dr. French's care and that we were interested in confirming his licensure, we were given information we never dreamed of receiving.

The man on the phone verified that Dr. French did have good credentials, adding "you are by no means the first persons to ask this question. As we speak, an investigation is being conducted by Dr. French's colleagues. This coming Monday morning they plan to place a complaint on Dr. French's desk stating their concerns."

Expecting to be stonewalled by bureaucratic evasion, we were astonished by the candor of this man. Taking the initiative, he asked how long my relatives had been clients of Dr. French. When we said it had been about ten years, his response was a simple, "Oh, my!" His next question came unexpectedly. "Do you have hard evidence of sexual misconduct by Dr. French?" He sounded disappointed we had none.

The information we gleaned from this spokesman assured us we had good reason to distrust Dr. French. It appeared clear to us that the state office had not only received numerous inquiries and complaints concerning Dr. French, but some of them had included sexual allegations.

Glaring inequites stood out in bold relief. Authorities needed some kind of hard evidence in order to establish Dr. French's guilt, even in the light of multiple testimonies against him. Yet *one lone accusation* against my father, without so much as a cursory search for any hard evidence, was enough for Dr. French to declare Dad's guilt. A blatantly different set of rules protected our lofty therapist.

Without prompting from us, the Mental Health spokesman voluntarily enumerated four facts he knew to be true about Dr. French.

"Number one," he said, "Dr. French is *very* Freudian."

This statement is categorically denied by his followers because Dr. French himself denies it. Yet this fellow psychologist told us that the mental health community in which Dr. French practiced considered him to be decidedly Freudian, a position deemed outmoded by his peers.

When my husband asked what he meant by saying Dr. French was *very* Freudian, the man responded, "Dr. French's answer is *always incest!*" Surprise turned to amazement! We had not yet told this person what our complaint was, yet he was already answering our unspoken questions!

"Number two," he continued, "Dr. French hates women!"

Ah, but my sisters considered him the most loving person on earth. I guess it depends on your perspective. They venerated at his feet and felt he loved them. I looked him in the eye and experienced his scorn.

The man on the phone had hit the target two times out of two, shooting blind. I wondered how long he could sustain such a record.

"Number three, Dr. French has a history of dividing families."

Bull's eye again! He had caused a division of Grand Canyon proportions in our family.

On point number four, I thought the man had finally missed his mark. I could understand his viewpoint because I was sure that it was generally true. But I hoped that we would prove him wrong because ours was, after all, a Christian family, brought up on strong Bible training and under the protection of parental prayers. So when he said, "Number four, logic from within the family will *never* work," I couldn't accept his verdict.

As I write this over a decade later, I admit that I have since acquiesced to his superior wisdom. I now understand why, when he learned our sisters had been under Dr. French's care for eight or ten years, he replied with a spontaneous, "Oh, my!" For at the time of this writing, neither logic, argument, prayer, patience, confrontation, nor unflattering national media exposure has made a discernable difference in my sisters' glowing opinions of Dr. French, nor in their embracing of his conclusions regarding their own father.

In spite of the fact that "logic from within the family" carries little weight, there are victims of this kind of psychological brainwashing who are "coming out" and retracting their accusations. They realize and acknowledge they have been duped and manipulated by their therapists. Someone, or something, *is* reaching them.

I hope someday someone will be able to help extricate our victims.

Chapter Five

Aftermath

Back in Ginny's car for the return trip from Dr. French's office, I was still reeling from the bomb dropped into my lap by my sister Lillian and her therapist. I wondered what I should say to Ginny, since I had been forbidden to tell anyone—especially my family—what they had revealed to me. But Ginny soon assured me that she already knew all the accusations Lillian had leveled against our father. Furthermore, she thought they must be true!

Again I struggled in a mental tug-of-war, wondering whether I was the only person alive who was living in the real world, or whether I had never even had a close encounter with reality myself. I felt as if I were flying an airplane without instruments, unable to tell if my plane had flipped upside down, or if my senses had just gone wacky.

Why did Ginny give credence to Lillian and Dr. French's portrayal of Dad, when it was diametrically opposed to everything she knew about our father? Was it so inconceivable for her to contradict the pronouncements of her guru? Was it because she was unable to believe Lillian had blatantly lied about our father? Could it be she found it impossible to think our younger sister could not distinguish between fact and fantasy? Assuming all the above were true, why, oh why was it so easy for her to discard Daddy's lifetime of integrity?

In spite of the fact that Ginny's actions made no sense to me, being made privy to the secret previously known only by these two sisters had produced a camaraderie with them not possible in recent years. I admit to a degree of headiness at being accepted into the "in crowd," much as a sorority candidate savors acceptance after a gruelling initiation.

Ginny filled me in on some details of Lillian's previous self-destructiveness and her inability to perform the simple routines of daily life. She voiced the question that also haunted me: "Wasn't it impossible to explain the wretchedness of Lillian's life without identifying some hideous devastation that had triggered it?"

How desperately I needed someone to help me gain perspective. How urgently I needed the counsel and wisdom of my level-headed husband. Who was this imposter/therapist who had put an uncrossable chasm between myself and my spouse? Behold how he divides families!

I wondered, "Do I have the right to disregard Dr. French's gag rule?" My inclination to do so was tempered by the fact that my oldest sister Anna seemed to be confident in Dr. French's ability, his integrity, and his apparent success in initiating some degree of healing in Lillian.

Anna was stable, discerning and credible. I found it incomprehensible that while she defended French, she never stated to me that she felt Dad was innocent of incest.

Years would pass before we could untangle the web of "who knew what and when" enough to discover that Anna knew very little of what Lillian and Dr. French had presented to me as fact. Anna based her conclusions regarding Dr. French on her confidence in the pastor who recommended him, on French's association with a well-reputed theological seminary, and more importantly, on her observation that Lillian seemed better able to cope with life after receiving some therapy than when she first came to the Northwest.

Aftermath

Anna expected that as Lillian continued to improve, Dr. French would eventually help her recognize her mistaken impression about her father. Accusations of incest were not known to Anna, nor could she have imagined that incest had become a consideration.

~

If in truth I had spent a portion of that day in the viper's den, that night I found myself in the regions of the damned. I felt stripped of my past, unable to comprehend my present, and terrified of my future. My mind vacillated between the certainty that Lillian was dead wrong, and the conviction that no one could invent such fallacy.

Alone and unable to sleep, I wondered what Dr. French and my sisters expected me to do with my new information. After all, I had been instructed to tell no one. I wasn't allowed to contradict them or refute their story. I could identify no plausible course of action I could take regarding it. I felt violated and abandoned, as if they had dumped a load of manure on me and then stripped me of any means to clean it up.

But something more than mere shock and confusion was at work here. In Dr. French's office I had felt—perhaps I should say I discerned—an unmistakable pressure to capitulate. Something outside myself was reasoning with me, attempting to coerce me to agree that Dr. French and Lillian's rendition of events in my life was the truth, in spite of what I knew to be true.

Though some might identify the force I felt to be a combination of peer pressure and a compulsion to submit to an authority figure, I am convinced it was more—much more—than that.

I believe that, stripped of all props and defenses, I stood exposed and vulnerable in the midst of an intense spiritual battle being waged over my ability to discern between truth and error. I believe that, had I capitulated to that coercive pressure by exchanging actual truth for their "false truth," I would have tipped the scales toward the disintegration of my personality—to insanity.

Skeletons Without Bones

Now that I know the full extent of Dr. French's debauchery, I am certain the force in that office I had hitherto been reluctant to identify was, in fact, demonic. The choice before me was whether I would hold fast to what I knew to be truth—and ultimately, Him whose name is Truth—or whether I would abandon truth and succumb to a lie, subsequently yielding ground to him who is the Father of Lies.

That night, in an effort to regain some semblance of mental equilibrium, I penned a letter to Lillian, still trying to maintain the precarious position that I accepted her explanations. I told her I was glad to have my little sister back, after years of estrangement. I admitted that her story presented an explanation for her condition consistent with current theories of psychology, and could seem to provide a key to understanding the puzzle that was Lillian.

Re-reading that letter some fourteen years later, I recoiled at the near-incoherency of my attempt to maintain common ground between us. Perhaps the letter's only real value was that it helped me endure the most intolerable night of my lifetime.

The following day my husband and I, along with our sons, left the great Northwest, headed for our next assignment.

Years before, we had purchased a GMC over-the-road coach which Gary had transformed into a two-bedroom motor home, complete with washer, dryer, a full bath and even a full-sized piano. As was our custom before an early morning departure, we made most of our necessary preparations the previous night. Next morning Gary did the final chores and took off while the boys and I remained asleep. It was an arrangement we all could appreciate.

Finally falling asleep in the early morning hours, I loathed to awaken that next morning to my altered world. But during that long night I had come to terms with Dr. French's restraints. He possessed no authority which allowed him to erect a barrier of that magnitude between my husband and me. I owed him neither allegiance nor deference.

Confident that the children would remain asleep for some time, I joined Gary at the front of the bus, ready to disgorge the entire unsavory mess.

Until that moment, I had told my husband only that I had learned Lillian had been sexually molested as a child. When he had asked by whom, I said, "I am not at liberty to say." He had not pressed me for details. He had no clue my father had been implicated and never suspected the intensity of my emotional upheaval.

With the panorama of the eastern slopes of the Cascade Mountains all about us as we topped the divide, I told my husband I was ready to tell him who had been named as Lillian's molester.

Gary looked at me expectantly—but I could go no further. I simply could not speak. The previous day I had spent several hours discussing with Dr. French and my two sisters their assumptions of Daddy's guilt. Now, beyond the sphere of their influence, I could not begin to repeat the story for my husband. "Telling" proved to be as difficult as "not telling."

Several times I ventured, "It was...." "It was...." I had intended to speak to Gary with the same dogmatic authority with which they had told me, thus passing on to him the full impact of the announcement. But I could not force the words out of my mouth. Seeing my struggle, Gary placed his hand on mine.

"Are you sure you want to tell me?"

Still mute, I nodded. "It was...."

Momentarily I panicked. Would Gary, like Ginny, give credence to Dr. French? What if he said, "I always *did* wonder about your father!"?

Finally I forced the words out. "It was my Daddy!"

Gary reacted as if he had been shot. Forever I will bless him for it, though for a moment I thought he might drive our bus into a ravine!

Just saying the words had left me in shambles. I buried my face in my hands, the sobs coming hard.

Gary's matter-of-fact question cut through my tears, putting starch back into my spine. "Are you *sure*?"

Ah, leave it to Gary to go to the heart of the matter. Of course I wasn't sure! I didn't even believe it. It was *they* who had been so sure. Dr. French had said, "We are giving you absolute facts. You can accept the truth, or you can remain forever a 'Pollyanna'."

Gary provided the stability of reason that I drastically needed. His clear-headedness served as a balm to my raw emotions, an anchor for my churning thoughts.

Gary waited for my answer. I shook my head. "No! Of course I'm not sure. But that is what they told me."

Gary was quiet for only a moment. Then he said with easy conviction, "I could believe it of myself before I could believe it of your dad."

"Thank you, Lord! And thank you, Gary! The whole world is *not* crazy! And neither am I!"

CHAPTER SIX

To the Accuser Belong the Spoils

Twenty-four hours after meeting with Dr. French and Lillian, I was hundreds of miles from the West Coast. In retrospect, I suspect Dr. French purposely planned our appointment to take place just prior to our time of departure.

Left now to my own devices, I vacillated between anger at having my father falsely accused, guilt for failing to declare his innocence, and shame for concluding my sister was a liar. But by the time two tortured weeks had gone by, I was anxious to tell Lillian that her "memories" were nothing more than figments of her imagination.

But how should I break the news to her? Should I be firm and tough, a-bristle with righteous indignation?—(I thought how an angry Jesus had thrown the moneychangers out of the temple.) Or should I be understanding and sympathetic, awash with long-suffering?—(I pictured a gentle Jesus restoring respectability by granting forgiveness to a wayward woman.) Whichever course I would choose to take, I felt sure that any contradiction of Lillian would have disastrous ramifications for us all.

Always before I had been able to find guidance and comfort from the Bible in times of distress. However, I now found myself unable to concentrate long enough to comprehend even a few verses of Scripture. I could only plead, "Lord, give me the right words and proper attitude toward my sister when I tell her the truth about what I believe."

That first Sunday morning back on the road, we were scheduled to sing and preach in a Church of the Nazarene in north central Montana. I privately wondered, "How can I—as nearly a basket case as I have ever seen—minister to others? I desperately need someone to minister to me!" But soon I marveled at the faithfulness of God to meet me at my place of need as my husband's sermon text spoke directly to me: "Fear not: believe only."[1]

Those simple words spoken by Jesus became life and breath to my suffering spirit. I had often wondered why Jesus spoke to broken people in such trite, simplistic terms. Why didn't He give them something meatier to chew, or something profound to ponder?

In that moment I understood. It is undistracted minds that are best suited for intellectual and spiritual pursuits. But Jesus knew a drowning man or woman needs a simple lifeline, not instructions for building a lifeboat. That pithy phrase, scaled to the limits of my current mental and emotional capacities, became my lifeline.

"Fear not: believe only." It bore its way through my spiritual fog and lodged itself firmly in my mind, easily comprehended and retained. Maybe I would never understand Lillian and her accusation, but I could choose to believe the Lord remained sovereign and that He was in control, even when it appeared otherwise.

I was given no mystical revelation that "our side wins." I received no assurance that Lillian would retract her accusations, or that Dad would be proven innocent, his name cleared. I had not been promised that my family would be healed and whole again. But I knew the Lord had spoken to me through his Word that "life did not end in Dr. French's office. God is not dead. We will get through this together. Do not be overwhelmed; trust me."

Thus strengthened and reassured, I began to plan how I would tell Lillian that there was absolutely no evidence anywhere that one particle of her story was true.

We had all grown accustomed to tiptoeing around Lillian, having been warned that because of her fragile emotional state, any challenge to her charges could trigger a suicide attempt. Whether she might have done so, I do not know. But I do know that Dr. French used the possibility of suicide to control our entire family and to quash any resistance or repudiation we might have raised.

So, in an attempt to avoid any such tragic consequences, I first wrote my repudiation of Lillian's story in a letter to Dr. French, giving him ample opportunity to provide for her emotional support if he so desired. Included in the letter was the following parable:

The Moon is round. All my life the Moon has been round.

But one day Dr. French informed me, "Donna, the Moon is not round. It is square. It attacked and hurt Lillian with its sharp corners. She has suffered from its cruelty. You must believe what we tell you. The Moon is square."

Lillian described to me how it felt to be attacked by a square Moon. She showed me her wounds. She asked, "Donna, do you believe me?"

I looked at Lillian. I saw her wounds. I said, "Lillian, I don't see how you could make up a story like that."

Again I looked at the Moon, this time with new information and with some suspicion. I said, "I KNOW Lillian would not lie. Could the Moon be square?"

But I have looked at the Moon. I have examined it intensely. No matter what you say—in spite of Lillian's "experience" and your evaluations, Dr. French—the Moon is not square.

The Moon is round.

Anxious to rid myself of my supportive role, I next phoned Ginny to tell her of my renunciation of the accusations against Dad.

To my surprise, Ginny responded to my defection with an unruffled, "I hope Lillian can accept the news without serious repercussions." But her next statement instantly raised my hackles: "Dr. French said we may never know for sure."

"*What did you say?*"

She repeated, "Dr. French said we may never know for sure."

I don't think I ever felt such rage!

"We may never know for sure?" What about Lillian's note to me with all the gory details of my father's violation of her? What about the "oral and rectal" part? Weren't these the memories that were supposed to be real, "whether I believed them or not?" Weren't they presented to me as positive proof of Dad's guilt?

"We may never know for sure?" Then where did these explicit details come from? Did they happen, or didn't they? Were they admitting among themselves that her memories could have been fabricated—hallucinations of a sick mind? What had happened to the indisputable facts they had thrust upon me?

How dare Dr. French label me a "Pollyanna" for rejecting a preposterous story he himself admitted could be false!

After my anger had waned, I was able to regard their spurious accusations in a different light. If, at the outset, I had in fact betrayed Dad by not openly contradicting their allegations, perhaps I had evened the score by repudiating their "facts" before I knew the flimsy construction of their square moon!

I have never again heard anyone allude to the idea, "we may never know for sure." It seems that fact has been stricken from the record since it only damages their hypothesis.

Playing fast and loose with truth seems to be what accusers and their supporters do best. When verifiable family facts fail to substantiate recovered memories, facts are readily discarded. Even when confronted with alternative conclusions, it is obvious that "therapists always did like repression best."

With Dr. French and Ginny now both aware of what I intended to do, I called to tell Lillian, "I do not believe your story about Dad. I concede that something horrible could have happened to you—maybe you have even been molested. I couldn't know that for sure.[2] But of one thing I am positive—you have suffered no harm from our father. I still love you and hope we can continue to have a friendly relationship, but it must be with the full knowledge that I disagree with your conclusions."

Surprisingly, she seemed able to accept me on those terms and we continued to interact with one another for some months after that.

Following a brief stay in Montana, my husband headed our motor home eastward toward Watertown, South Dakota where Al and Barb Wagner pastored the Wesleyan Church. Al and Barb made an outstanding pastoral team and were some of our dearest friends. They had often engaged us to conduct special services at the churches they served.

Unusually sensitive to the needs of others and gifted to minister to those needs, the Wagner home was the perfect place for me. The realization that the Lord had pre-arranged our schedule reminded me again to "fear not; believe only."

Barb became my confidante and provided much-appreciated emotional support. She agreed that Dr. French had no right to dump on me his interpretation of my family and then forbid me to seek counsel concerning his catastrophic allegations.

Barb felt I needed to talk to someone with intimate knowledge of my family some twenty-five years before—someone who could help me understand the discrepancy between Lillian's memories of our family and my own.

One couple met those qualifications—Mitchell and Angela Scott, our pastors in Deanton, Indiana.

Back in January of 1957, our denomination's international headquarters building in Syracuse, New York had burned to the ground. Rather than rebuild on the restricted site of the ancient building,

Skeletons Without Bones

church officials decided to relocate in Indiana. Employed as a foreman in the Publishing Department, Daddy had committed to go with the company, so we prepared to sell our house and move west to the Hoosier State.

Dad went to Indiana while Mom went to prayer. The law forbade removal of foster children from one state to another and she could not entertain the thought of going without her children. The State of New York unwittingly became the answer to her prayer by taking the matter to court and requesting that Mom and Dad be awarded legal guardianship of our foster children.

With the outcome of house and children still pending, Dad and my brother Peter went ahead to Indiana to help get the presses up and running and to find housing for us. Mother remained behind until we children finished out the school year in Syracuse.

Dad's primary concerns included more than just physical provision for his brood. Together he and Peter scouted local churches each Sunday morning and evening and again on Wednesday evening in search of a church home. Peter rejected each one until the night they heard Rev. Scott preach, and afterwards visited with him and his wife. Peter proposed, "I think we have found the church we are looking for." Dad agreed. So Dad bought a house within walking distance of that little church in Deanton, Indiana.

Not long out of college, Mitchell and Angela welcomed a seasoned pastor and Bible teacher into their fellowship. Soon Dad was leading the mid-week service and teaching Sunday school. Lillian became the favorite baby sitter for the Scott's two small children.

Mother often teased that Daddy's preliminary move to Indiana and his subsequent weekend visits back to Syracuse resulted in her late-in-life pregnancy. That first year in Deanton found us awaiting the birth of our little "Tag-along." Terry Lee arrived in March of 1958 when Mother was forty-nine years old, Dad was fifty-seven, and I was two months from high school graduation.

Already uneasy about this pregnancy, when miscarriage threatened, Dr. Arthur McIlroy ordered Mother to bed for the duration.

When Mom delivered, Dr. McIlroy was alarmed by the size and shape of the infant's head. His diagnosis was hydrocephalus—fluid on the brain. At three months Terry was still unable to hold his head up or sleep a night through. Dr. McIlroy was certain that Terry Lee had a serious disability.

In the wee hours one Friday night Angela Scott woke her husband. "Mitchell, the Lord is telling me we need to pray for McGraw's baby." So the pastor whom Peter and Dad had carefully chosen a few months previous knelt before the Lord, interceding on behalf of Daddy's newborn. They continued in prayer until Angela declared, "We can quit now. The Lord has healed Terry Lee."

That same night, Mother kept her usual vigil caring for a fretting baby. Suddenly he sat up straight, looked around in every direction, then settled down contentedly to sleep the night through. Later comparisons confirmed the Scotts' prayer time coincided exactly with Terry's unprecedented response.

The next morning Terry held his head up as if he had always done so. When Lillian encountered Mrs. Scott uptown the next morning, the lady confidently asked, "How is Terry? He's all right now, isn't he?"

Lillian agreed, "He appears to be much improved."

The following day at church, when Dad carried Terry to our family's unofficial pew—middle section, second row from the front—the other worshippers whispered to one another, "Look at McGraw's baby! He's holding his head up and looking around!"

Rev. Scott took Terry Lee to the platform. Holding aloft an alert infant, the pastor told of his wife's early morning call to prayer and of her assurance that the Lord had answered. There were no dissenters—only believers—in the wide-eyed congregation.

Because of their close relationship with our family, I considered the Scotts well-qualified to evaluate Lillian's accusations. Though I had not had direct contact with them since they left Deanton two years after Terry's healing some twenty years before, I still trusted their judgment, their knowledge and their spiritual discernment. I also knew they would tell me the unvarnished truth.

Skeletons Without Bones

A phone call to a distant state found them both at home. I described to them my recent experience in Dr. French's office, and asked, "Mitchell and Angela, Dr. French said it was the truth, whether I accepted it or not. Do I have to believe him?"

Still fresh in my memory is their swift and firm reassurance. "No, it is not true and you certainly do not have to believe it. Your father was a godly man and he became our class leader.[3] We would have known if something had been amiss."

Mitchell, not quite satisfied with the information I had given, questioned me further. "Donna, I sense there is something else, a piece missing from the puzzle. Can you think of anything else?"

There was, in fact, one thing I felt might be important. During Lillian's college years, her perfectionism concerning grades had constrained her to study and prepare for classes well into the night. She confessed to Gary and me that in order to keep alert, she had taken pep pills. When she would finally lay aside her books, too wired for natural rest, she took sleeping pills to induce sleep. I do not know how often she repeated that procedure but apparently it was her *modus operandi* throughout her college years.

That additional information put things in perspective for Mitchell. He had counseled many young people who had resorted to using drugs—either illegal or over-the-counter—as a coping mechanism. He had observed that the use of such chemical substances sometimes wiped out the real memories which make up a person's past. The resultant confusion often prompted the individual to seek counseling.

This explanation from Mitchell corresponded with my own suspicions and gave a logical explanation for Lillian's condition.

Given that Lillian's therapist had granted "most favored notion" status to the repression of memories of sexual abuse, he would readily conclude that Lillian had repressed a past too horrible to contemplate. The ensuing therapy would relentlessly lead her to discover the counselor's presuppositions.

The loving support I received from Mitchell and Angela Scott helped quell that question which, like a pesky weed, repeatedly sprang up in spite of myself: "Am I crazy?"

To the Accuser Belong the Spoils

When Lillian later discovered I had confided in the Scotts, she was angry because she had intended to call them to tell *her* story. She felt I had preempted her opportunity by getting to them first.

Thus I received one of my early lessons that "to the accuser belong the spoils." In the world of recovered repressed memories, countless boundaries and restrictions are established, multitudes of taboos and denied privileges are enforced. But these constraints are applied, not to the accusers, but to the accused, and to anyone else who doesn't buy into the allegations of the victim and her mentor.

The whole world belongs to accusers. They can say anything they please, and everything they say is considered gospel. They may change their story, contradict themselves and give obviously erroneous information. Any discrepancy is chalked up as the normal behavior of a poor, distraught victim.

On the other hand, no word from the accused or his supporters is given an ounce of credence. We are considered defensive and "Pollyannas," enablers hobbled by our own deposits of grotesque repressions. Any defense of the accused is construed as additional abuse heaped upon the poor victim, i.e., the accuser!

Few frustrations approach that of finding oneself totally erased, credited with no significance, and possessing no validity—discovering that in the world of recovered repressed memories, "to the accuser belong the spoils."

CHAPTER SEVEN

"In the Mouth of Two or Three Witnesses"

Mitchell and Angela Scott took me one step closer toward regaining emotional equilibrium by reassuring me I had not lost my sanity.

But there could be no joy in knowing my younger sister had adopted for herself an identity that was the figment of demented imaginations. Whether she was mistaken, misled, or deliberately malicious, her poison was communicable and she was adept at spreading it. A significant segment of my family already suffered from years of ingesting megadoses of her toxin. Unchecked, the damage would only proliferate.

If I remained silent, I would join the burgeoning ranks of individuals our society calls enablers, i.e., perpetrators of existing problems. On the other hand, by speaking out I would become a hated whistle-blower, creating a plethora of pitfalls of unknowable proportions and consequences to my loved ones.

Whether in wisdom or cowardice, I chose not to immediately disturb the *status quo*. As long as my parents remained in the Caribbean, I did not have to worry that they would be confronted with accusations. And I felt safe to assume my sister was unlikely to risk confiding in another family member any time soon.

Choosing not to reveal my experience to my family at this time did not prevent me from embarking upon my own investigation. I intended to hold in my hand some kind of evidence before it became necessary to "tell all."

Our family doctor back in Indiana seemed a reasonable person with whom to begin my search. He had seen all the McGraws as patients. He had attended Mother through her risky pregnancy and had delivered my brother Terry Lee. He had done the prenuptial blood testing for members of our family who had married while we lived in Indiana.

Most importantly, he had treated Lillian for menstrual difficulties during her early teens. A thorough physical exam would no doubt have been a routine part of his diagnosis.

No longer a small-town practitioner at the time I made my inquiry, Dr. McIlroy had become a resident physician on the staff of a nearby hospital. On March 12, 1981, the switchboard put me through to his office, and wonder of wonders, a voice answered, "Dr. McIlroy speaking."

I introduced myself and asked, "At your convenience, may I ask you some questions regarding my family as you knew them some years ago?" He surprised me by saying, "I would be glad to talk to you now as I eat my lunch in my office."

Briefly I told him of Lillian's recent accusations against my dad. "Dr. McIlroy, I do not for a moment believe her accusations are true. In your examinations of Lillian, did you encounter anything that aroused your suspicions? Would you have anything in your files indicating you had noticed anything amiss?"

As had been true in the case of the Scotts, Dr. McIlroy's reply came swift and firm. "I have no need to consult my files. Your parents were guardians of foster children. Had I entertained the slightest question, I was obligated by law to report it to the authorities. I assure you, I would not have hesitated to do so."

He further stated, "Your mother was one of the most natural-born mothers I have ever known."

How different were the opinions expressed by people who knew my parents, as opposed to the wild theories of one ignorant, prejudiced psychologist!

Dr. McIlroy followed his affirmation with his own disclosure.

"It's funny you should ask me these questions. Lillian herself wrote me a couple of years ago asking essentially the same thing. I remember it well because I had never received a letter so full of bitterness and anger as was that one."

He continued, "I don't like to use the word 'charlatan' but I strongly advised her to get a second opinion from another therapist."

Once again I struggled with outrage at the unmitigated deception that had been heaped upon me. An iron-clad case against my dad? Hardly!

A child who had experienced what Lillian's note indicated would have had physical indications. If Dr. McIlroy had been obligated to report suspected irregularities, so would the doctors in New York State who had seen her in childhood and pre-teen years. Those same doctors would have attended both the natural-born and foster children in our home. Would those health care professionals have overlooked signs of child abuse? I dare say, "No, of course not." They, like Dr. McIlroy, would not have hesitated to report their suspicions.

Lillian had not told me that Dr. McIlroy had advised to her to seek a second opinion, another example of how information is selectively chosen when building a case for long-forgotten sexual abuse. If a piece of the puzzle cannot be twisted and reshaped to fit its predetermined spot, it is simply discarded, deemed unworthy of consideration.

Dr. McIlroy expressed doubt that our family had any recourse in dealing with Dr. French. But he advised us to make sure his credentials were in order and told us how to do so.

Before concluding our conversation, Dr. McIlroy asked, "Whatever happened to your baby brother I delivered?"

I told him, "Terry attended college in Oklahoma before moving to California where he married and settled...." The doctor interrupted me.

"*COLLEGE? Terry went to COLLEGE?*"

Since that news rendered him speechless, I filled the silence for him. "Terry learned to read before he went to school. Mrs. Pattison—you remember the kindergarten teacher?—she had him read stories to the entire class to keep him occupied and to entertain and inspire the other children."

The usually articulate doctor was stuttering.

"I...I remember when...When I delivered him, I diagnosed him...I was sure he was hydrocephalic. He...he went to college? You say he was normal?"

With typical sibling sarcasm, I corrected him.

"I didn't say he was *normal*. I said he went to college."

He was too incredulous to appreciate my humor.

"Yes, Dr. McIlroy. Do you remember Pastor Mitchell and Angela Scott?" He remembered. He had been their doctor also.

I told him of their midnight prayer vigil and the subsequent miracle of Terry's healing.

He responded with, "Something happened, all right! I considered him not much more than a vegetable when he was born. And you say he went to college!"

That phone conversation ended with both of us equally stunned but gratified with what we had learned.

Following Dr. McIlroy's advice, the next day my husband and I placed a call to the governmental agency with oversight of licensing mental health professionals in the State of Washington. I believe it was called the Office of Mental Health, Drug Abuse and Alcoholism, located within the Department of Social and Health Services. The agency has since been restructured and that function now falls within the jurisdiction of the Department of Health in Olympia.

My husband and I took careful notes of the conversations we had with staff from that office, the substance of which appears in Chapter Four of this book. When we shared that information in letters to members of my family, some of them were offended by our statements and questioned their veracity. However, we possess the original notes taken during that exchange, including permission given us by the spokesman to quote him and use his name.

As for Dr. McIlroy's statements contained in this account, he has read the entire manuscript and given his approval. He even suggested his pseudonym used herein.

Our file was growing fat with confirmations of my parents' integrity, and with suspicions of the questionable methods and conclusions of Dr. French. Rev. and Mrs. Scott, Dr. McIlroy, and now the spokesman for the Mental Health Office in Washington State all had provided valuable input.

Whether the information would ever help restore order to a family in chaos, I could not tell.

Chapter Eight

The Man I Call Daddy!

I hope I am accurate in making the following evaluation of my own motives: I include this chapter about my father not merely to vindicate him. Rather, my basic intent is to show how a therapist, by applying internal bias to information given by a client, may erroneously interpret the actions, character and behavior—even the thoughts and motives—of a third party that the therapist has never met.

To a client already mesmerized by the wisdom, validation and unconditional love of her counselor, this reinterpretation of persons and events becomes tantamount to divine revelation, and effectively exempts the client from taking responsibility for the problems that prompted her to seek help. She, or he, then becomes an accomplice to the therapist by supplying more and more fodder to be digested by the therapist, later to be regurgitated for assimilation by the client!

I portray my father as a man of exceptional morals and integrity, not only because he was such a man, but to underscore an important fact: if a therapist could twist my whistle-clean father into a predatory, Bible-wresting pedophile, what chance remains for any accused man to defend his innocence? This becomes especially germane if an accused man's daughter can in truth cite her father's outbursts of anger, his penchant for girly magazines, or his over-indulgence in alcoholic beverages. If my parents were not immune, no human being is safe, and therein lies the seriousness of the problem.

So I indulge in biographical accounts of my parents, as well as of my sister and her psychologist, to demonstrate how irresponsible methods are used by arrogant professionals to arrive at foolish, catastrophically damaging conclusions.

Christmas Eve, 1899, Jenny and Jacob McGraw of rural Breezewood, Pennsylvania, welcomed their eighth and last child whom they named John Edwin.

Dad's sister Pearl liked to tell us children how they had spoiled their baby brother, the youngest child by six years. One of her favorite stories told of young John sulking because he had to carry water to his brothers working in the harvest fields.

John left his play to fill the bucket at the pump and lug it out to the field. He handed the dipper to his brother, who filled it with the welcome refreshment. Only after Earl drained it dry did John confess with sweet revenge, "I 'tuck my dirty fin'er in it!"

We don't know much of Daddy's early years. We do know that as a young man, measuring six foot one and "skinny as a rail" at the onset of World War I, he was rejected for military service because the physical exam determined he was underweight, flat-footed and susceptible to ear infections. In those days before antibiotics, ear infections often resulted in complications for which the United States military was not anxious to assume responsibility.

The Man I Call Daddy!

Dad was thirteen years old when his father died. His mother died not many years later. Dad and his brother Earl went to live with their oldest sister in Pittsburgh. There Dad at age eighteen attended a gospel meeting at Everybody's Mission, which resulted in his Christian conversion. Whatever had been his goals prior to that experience, they were put to rest as he set his sights on living under the leadership of the Lord. As far as I know, he never wavered from that commitment.

Often expressing himself in poetry, on the fiftieth anniversary of his conversion, Dad wrote:

> *Just fifty years ago today*
> > *Christ washed my every sin away.*
> *Repentant to the throne I came,*
> > *And trusted in the Savior's name.*
> *The Lamb of God for me had died,*
> > *Had shed his blood through riven side;*
> *In looking to that crimson tide*
> > *My soul was fully justified.*
> *Redeeming blood paid every debt.*
> > *Redeeming blood let God forget.*
> > *Redeeming blood—My refuge yet!*
>
> *The Spirit's witness was so clear*
> > *It banished every doubt and fear.*
> *By the new life God's love bestowed*
> > *I changed from broad to narrow road.*
> *Brought back from mountain bleak and cold,*
> > *The Shepherd led me to his fold.*
> *That there could never be a doubt,*
> > *Adoption papers were made out.*
> *So I became a LEGAL heir,*
> > *And joined with Christ, a REGAL heir,*
> > *To mansions He went to prepare.*
>
> *There has been, will be, storm and stress,*

Skeletons Without Bones

> *When Satan's hosts so sorely press;*
> *But anchored safe within the vail*
> *Where Jesus is, I need not fail.*
> *With penitential attitude,*
> *With faith and hope and vows renewed,*
> *By Holy Spirit power endued,*
> *The years, now past, have been reviewed!*
> *E'er fifty more years flee apace*
> *I'll see my Savior face to face—*
> *"And tell the story saved by Grace."*

Following that life-changing event, John enrolled in God's Bible School in Cincinnati, Ohio. Fred Messer, a fellow student and friend, told Dad about the need for pastors in Oklahoma and Texas. Upon completion of his studies, Dad made his way southwest where he was given an assignment within the Oklahoma Conference of The Wesleyan Methodist Connection.

Dad's second assignment was to start a church in a rural community near the town of Alva. He began holding Sunday services in the local schoolhouse where he taught during the week. Later, pastor and people erected a building called simply "Cedar Grove Church."

To this church Daddy brought his bride Amy of Alton, Kansas. To that union were born two daughters, Anna and Louise, and a son, John E. McGraw, Jr. Born a "blue baby," Daddy's firstborn son lived only a few short hours.

More tragedy was in store for the little parsonage family. With child for the fourth time, Amy soon discovered something was amiss. The family made hasty preparations to rush her to town to the doctor.

But an early January thaw had caused the frost to go out of the ground, turning those old dirt roads into impassable mires of sticky clay. Suffering a tubal pregnancy and isolated from medical assistance, Amy's young life came to a sudden end.

The grieving pastor cared for his young daughters with the help of the ladies of the church. The girls also spent time with their maternal grandparents of rural Alton.

The Man I Call Daddy!

About one year following Amy's death, Dad set his heart on winning the hand of Opal Cummings of Enid, Oklahoma. An acquaintance of both John and Amy, Opal often sang in churches around that area.

They courted primarily by correspondence. The original letters, yellowed and fragile, remain in my possession, a legacy of their love and anticipation of marriage.

The last of the letters written in my father's fluid script bears the date April 29, 1933. Less than a week before their wedding, he wrote:

> *Opal, the name you are about to take upon you, while not of earthly greatness, is one you need not be ashamed of. My home was not as spiritual as yours, but it was a good home. Its influence and that of the Spirit and Word of God kept me from that which would be of special regret at this time.*
>
> *Never once have you cheapened in any way yourself in my eyes. Never once have I lowered the very high estimation that I have had of your wonderful character. You have been a perfect lady. And as my wife, I promise you that you shall have every consideration and right that belongs to you. I shall endeavor not to fall below your estimation of a gentleman.*

So Daddy won a new bride and a new mother for his two little girls, now six and four years old. Both girls attest to the ease with which Opal stepped into the role of mother to her ready-made family.

Before long the family found itself preparing for another blessed event. Not far into the pregnancy Mother's appendix ruptured, necessitating an emergency appendectomy. It is easy to imagine Daddy's concern as he again faced uncertainties regarding his wife and unborn child.

Both mother and child weathered the surgery and Virginia arrived at the proper time, hale and hearty. No one guessed she would cry with the colic for six weeks solid!

Skeletons Without Bones

During the next ten years, Dad pastored several rural churches throughout Oklahoma and Texas. Meanwhile, the family expanded as Mildred, Peter, Donna and Lillian followed at two and three year intervals.

Both Lillian and I were born while the family lived in a little three-room parsonage beside New Hope Church near Ringwood, Oklahoma. Actually, the house was composed of two rooms, with a lean-to fastened on the back to provide desperately needed sleeping room. Child number six, I am told my first bed was a dresser drawer. Typically I respond: "Yes, and Millie kept closing the drawer on me."

My earliest memory was formed at New Hope—a fuzzy mental picture of our entire family sleeping outdoors on old-fashioned iron bedsteads. The four corner bedposts punctured the bare, sandy soil littered with a healthy crop of annoying sandburrs. Our house stood as a backdrop nearby, stars stabbing holes in the black canopy overhead.

We slept several persons to a bed, which was normal for us. I remember the soothing sound of my father's voice coming from somewhere across the yard. I don't recall what he said but it seemed somehow connected with looking at the stars overhead.

I cherished that memory, for it held for me all the warmth and security of family intimacy. I felt no fear, though it was dark and I was only two or three.

As I grew older, reason chided me that when you sleep outside, it is not on a bed but rather on the ground. I reluctantly reclassified my memory as a pleasant dream. Then one day I overheard my sister Millie telling a friend that when we lived at New Hope, the summer nights were stifling as we slept nine persons in our cramped little house. In search of much-needed air, we carried our beds outside and slept in the yard!

I recognized her story as the fleshing out of my discarded memory! And it would be typical of my Dad to take advantage of the star-studded sky visible overhead to talk of God's wonderful creation and His special care for each of us.

That earliest of my memories epitomizes my concept of my family. We belonged together and we liked being together. At the helm, Dad provided stability and purpose, guiding without forcing, steering a steady course through every storm. Mom, the unharried nurturer, calmly enjoyed the chaos that whirled around her as she mothered her boisterous brood in perpetually cramped quarters.

People who knew Dad only slightly thought him to be stern. He did have a serious nature and was basically shy, not totally at ease in strictly social settings. He never really mastered the art of polite small talk, and societal amenities bored him.

Dad's commonness belied his intellectual prowess. He was without pomp, airs or pretense and was not impressed by such characteristics in others. Easily overlooked in a crowd of important-looking persons, Dad astounded men of learning if they chanced to engage him in conversation.

This fact was confirmed to our older son during his first year of college. The philosophy professor, whom Dustin had already labeled his most intellectual instructor, surprised Dustin by saying, "I know your Grandfather McGraw. I had no idea that timid pastor I had seen at conference had such a wealth of knowledge until we made a cross-country trip to General Conference together."

At another ministerial gathering, some pastors asked our highest denominational official who he considered to be the best sermonizer in the organization. Dr. Roy S. Nicholson at first declined to make such a judgment. When his interrogators persisted, Dr. Nicholson named my father, stating, "John McGraw can craft a worthy sermon outline from nearly any passage of Scripture."

Dad thought in the context of sermon outlines. As a young pastor driving truck on the Martin farm during wheat harvest, Dad's sermon-writing propensities were legendary. For years those old farm trucks bore mute evidence, for all available surfaces on doors, dashboard and visors were inscribed with sermon outlines, complete with Scripture references. Lack of desk and paper was not sufficient deterrent to quell the churning-out of sermon material from Dad's fertile mind.

Skeletons Without Bones

My best friend in seventh grade said it all as she left our house one evening after school, "Doesn't your father do anything but read and write?"

With as much surprise as she had shown, I countered, "What in the world does *your* father do?"

She said, "He lies on the couch, drinking beer and watching TV." It was impossible to imagine my father in that context! I began to suspect maybe we weren't entirely typical.

As serious minded as he was, Dad was not without a quick wit and a keen sense of humor. By the time Terry Lee was a young buck in his late teens, Dad had lived three-quarters of a century. One day Terry asked, "Dad, how old does a man get before he loses interest in sex?" Dad looked at his young son, his blue eyes twinkling, and with a shrug of his shoulders, replied, "I don't know, Terry. Sometime after seventy-five."

A gentle man, Dad demonstrated infinite patience with his children, except when he was trying to corral them into the car to get to church on time. We usually had depleted his store of longsuffering long before we all piled in. And then invariably someone had forgotten a Bible or Mother discovered she was without dentures. Whenever another licensed driver was available, Dad opted to walk to church, leaving the last-minute hassle to less organized mortals.

The early riser of the family, Dad made his own breakfast. If he found dishes in the sink from the night before, he often washed them in the pre-dawn hours so they wouldn't be left for Mother that morning.

Knowing his early routine, we children loved to play tricks on Dad. When there were hard-cooked eggs to put away after supper, we would mix them back into the carton with the uncooked ones, hoping Dad would pick a cooked one to fry for his breakfast. We speculated that after two or three tries, he would expect yet another hard one, ensuring a culinary disaster when he used unwarranted force to crack a fragile raw egg.

Another of our ploys stemmed from Daddy's custom of taking a drink of water and leaving his glass upside down on the counter for his later use. Sometimes at night we would fill his glass with water, cover it with paper, quickly up-end the glass on the counter and carefully pull out the paper. We hoped Dad would meet his own Waterloo when he picked up the glass the following morning.

I don't remember Dad alluding to our antics on his own initiative, or reprimanding us for our bothersome pranks. But if asked about it, he just grinned his grin, and acted as if nothing at all had happened.

Sunday afternoons were designated as times of rest and quietness at our house in observance of the Lord's Day. If we kids didn't actually nap, we were expected to read or play quietly, giving Mom and Dad a chance to sleep.

One particular Sunday afternoon, a minor incident accelerated into an "act of terror" which has become a personal favorite.

Our parents' room stood at the top of the uncarpeted stairwell in our home in Syracuse. Near the bottom, the staircase made a right-angle turn, with a railing of upright posts separating the landing from the hardwood floor of the living room. Located below the landing was the hot-air register over which Dad often knelt in prayer on chilly mornings.

This typically tranquil Sunday afternoon found us playing with the marbles. Passed along from child to child, by the time I was nine or ten, our marble collection had multiplied to an amalgamation of sizes and colors that filled one large oatmeal box and one small one.

I think it was Lillian who helped carry the containers full of marbles from our upstairs bedroom as we made our way downstairs. En route a couple of marbles rolled over the edge of the box, through the railing which separated the upstairs hallway from the stairwell, over the precipice, and down the remaining steps.

For such little fellows, they made an amazing racket in the Sunday stillness. Eyes wide and hands over our mouths, we waited to see if we had wakened our parents. Hearing no reprimand reminding us to be quiet, we began to giggle over our inadvertent noise-making.

From that humble beginning a great plan took shape. What if we were to tip over both boxes at the top of the staircase, causing all the marbles to roll down the entire flight?

We developed our strategy. After we set the marbles rolling, we would run for our lives. That way no one would know who the culprits were, thus delaying and perhaps averting negative consequences. It sounded like just the sort of excitement needed to spice up a languishing Sunday afternoon.

Accordingly, we knelt at the top of the staircase, slowly tilting our boxes. In our wildest dreams we could not have anticipated the din that ensued as the noise of those two pilot marbles multiplied a thousand times.

Freed from captivity, the more ambitious marbles took off lickety-split and did a high jump off the first step, taking the whole flight in only two or three bounces. They leaped the landing, struck the floor on a dead run, maneuvered past the grid of the register and careened across the living room, where they ricocheted off the far wall to coast to a reluctant standstill somewhere mid-living room.

Other marbles opted for a more leisurely descent. Meandering to the stair's edge, they dropped to the first step and bounced a little staccato dance before gravity pulled them to the next level where they repeated their performance down the entire flight.

Our best shooters proved themselves Super-Marbles by leaping over the entire melee in a single bound, then muscling past their companions before bowing out to disappear beneath the sofa. Smaller, less fortunate glassies made an impressive descent but never made it across the hot air register. They could be heard reluctantly clunking their way through a mysterious labyrinth of metal heat ducts to destinations unknown, never to be heard from again.

Our well-laid plan of escape collapsed as we realized no one could descend that staircase and live. We remained riveted to the spot, dumbstruck at the longevity of our antics. Daddy yelled something that sounded like, "What on earth is going on?", but his words were drowned out by the thunderous noise of multitudes of marbles still cavorting down the stairwell.

An eternity had passed since we had propelled the first marbles over the edge but the fiasco gave no signs of letting up. Unwary marbles that had petered out were leaped upon by more aggressive comrades still on the attack. Together they searched out immobile cohorts, goading them back into the fray.

By now Dad had burst through his bedroom door, adrenalin pumping, poised for either fight or flight. It was the first and last time I ever saw my modest father clad only in his underwear. I had expected to be soundly reprimanded, and justly so, for my little practical joke had burgeoned into a huge breach of Sunday protocol.

However, one look at Dad's face told me that if the ensuing commotion had taken me unaware, my surprise could not begin to rival Dad's absolute terror at being jolted from his nap by a pandemonium of immense proportions and impossible identification reverberating throughout his entire house. To add to the mayhem, by now everyone within hearing distance—and that was a considerable range—both inside and outside the house had come on a dead run, yelling, "What happened? What is going on?"

Marbles were *still* bouncing and rolling. I feared we had just invented perpetual motion. The furnace ducts rumbled like caverns full of demons. Rescuers who heroically came dashing into the front room or the adjoining dining room were predestined to be unceremoniously catapulted into the midst of the fracas. Lillian and I stood trapped at the scene of the crime at the top of the staircase, dreading sentencing.

Daddy had by now had time to assess the situation as he viewed two wide-eyed little girls clutching empty oatmeal boxes, marbles everywhere. His terror gave way to relief as he discovered the bedlam had been caused, not by natural disaster or personal catastrophe, but by two kids playing with marbles. His familiar grin appeared, quickly extinguished by the astonished realization, akin to that of Adam's in Eden, that he was not properly clothed.

He never bothered to remind us to pick up our mess as, like Adam, he hid himself behind the closest shelter—in this case, the

Skeletons Without Bones

bedroom door. I can only imagine him describing the scene to Mother.

Having caught his grin, I dared survey the chaos with the satisfaction of a mission accomplished, admittedly with a degree of overkill.

The incident birthed a "family tradition." We knew better than to push our luck too often, but occasionally we would see the marbles and find ourselves unable to resist the urge to re-enact our crime. However, we were wiser now. We carefully closed the door at the bottom of the stairwell so the marbles would be corralled before they hit the landing and scattered to the four winds. Although Dad never again came bounding out in his shorts, the re-enactment never failed to liven up an all-too-serene Sunday afternoon. And Dad never lost his sense of humor over the antics of his mischievous offspring.

This incident illustrates the warmth, congeniality and interaction of our home. It was a hilarious place to grow up. Our friends loved to come over, sometimes voicing their envy at the "Cheaper by the Dozen"[1] atmosphere that prevailed there. Money and "nice things" were sometimes missing but they were not generally missed. Our wonderful Daddy was an integral part of the fun.

Maintaining a good-natured sense of humor was only one of Daddy's strong points. Though definitely not the touchy-feely type, he loved his kids and made untold sacrifices for their benefit.

I have described our move from New York State to Indiana when Dad's place of employment changed location following a devastating fire. I have also told how the New York State Welfare Department paid the court costs in order that the foster children under our care could be released to my parents rather than be uprooted and sent to new foster homes.

For caring for the children, Mother had received a monthly check from which she met her household expenses, thus making a substantial contribution to the family income. In addition, the State of New York had been responsible for the children's medical and dental expenses and all their clothing needs.

Following our move to Indiana, all that was changed. Daddy's income had to cover *all* the expenses. Mathematically, there was no way we could make it. In spite of that fact, there was no consideration by my parents of "whether" we would keep the children. It was only a matter of "how" the Lord would somehow make up the difference.

One tragedy resulted from that move to Indiana which almost destroyed my mother. My parents did not technically become legal guardians of the youngest of the four foster children. Eddie was a two-year-old Native American whom we had cared for since birth. His mother, a beautiful Onondaga Indian girl not yet twenty, spent every Sunday afternoon at our home with her son. Although her circumstances prevented her from raising him, she loved him and cherished the time she spent with him. Mother soon gained the confidence of this shy young woman, and Alice, too, fell heir to the mothering that came so easily to Mom.

When Alice learned we would be moving to a distant state, she agonized over her dilemma. How could she sign over to my parents the rights to her son, knowing she might never see him again? Yet, should she risk the impact that would follow if he were placed in another foster home?

She finally decided she would not sign over legal guardianship but she would allow Eddie to remain with us when we moved away. Though not an ideal arrangement, all parties agreed to it for want of a better solution.

The packers had worked most of the day getting the moving van filled and on its way. The younger children were put to bed, their traveling clothes and a favorite toy ready for an early departure for our new home in the Hoosier State.

About ten-thirty that evening a knock at the door revealed Alice standing on the porch. "I just can't bear to let Eddie go. My boy friend and I have decided to get married and make a home for my son."

With no opportunity for proper goodbyes, my stunned mother sadly watched as Alice took the sleeping toddler from his bed, picked up the meager bundle of his remaining possessions, and bade us farewell.

In a few minutes it was all over. For the second time in as many years Mother experienced the wrenching of a cherished child from her arms and heart.

A morbid group set out for points west the following morning. We each suffered our private losses of friends and loved ones. Entering a new school for my senior year threatened my early demise. But the knowledge that one of us was missing caused most of the tears that fell as we migrated to Indiana.

But this chapter is about Dad. We knew Mother's heart was broken at losing Eddie but Daddy's emotions were more difficult to read. After all, he did not know how he was going to support his additional dependents anyway. Was his sorrow mixed with some relief?

I found the answer to that question a few months later. By that time the pinch of diminished finances had increased to a stranglehold. In addition, the expenses of a risky pregnancy and a new baby now loomed on the horizon.

Into the midst of this scenario arrived a disturbing letter from Alice back in Syracuse.

> *I made a mistake in keeping Eddie. He cries constantly, looking everywhere for his mama and his brothers and sisters. He won't be comforted and I can't handle him. If you will come and get him, I promise never to interfere again other than by keeping in touch by letters and phone. How soon can you come?*

What could Mother say? She was without resources and she was pregnant! Dr. McIlroy had ordered her to bed. Unable to care for her household and uncertain of the future, it seemed unconscionable to even consider taking an additional child.

The long-range outlook proved no brighter since Mother could no longer augment the family income as she had in New York State. Besides, what would prevent Alice from changing her mind again?

The Man I Call Daddy!

Mom understood how difficult it would be for Alice to give up her child a second time.

But could she, should she, refuse to take Eddie back? We still had no solutions when a phone call came from a distraught Alice.

"Aren't you going to come get Eddie?"

Mother responded to this crisis as she had many others. She prayed. "Lord, if you want me to take Eddie, you will have to make me well and strong enough to make the trip to get him, and then to care for him and the rest of my children." Without further ado, she left her sick bed and never returned to it throughout the entire pregnancy.

I'll never forget that next Friday evening when Dad came home from work. He walked into the house and with his hand extended, he went straight to Mother. He put his entire week's paycheck into her hand and said, "Opal, you'd better go get our boy." Knowing the unspeakable circumstances under which Eddie was now living, Daddy had put reason and expediency aside to let his heart and his unshakable faith in the Lord's provision rule the day. To this moment I cannot recall that event with dry eyes.

This is the man who was my Daddy. Was he a selfish pervert who would violate his little daughter for his own warped gratification? A thousand times *NO*! What *hogwash*! He was a man who gave beyond his ability to give, in order to provide a chance for life to a child he loved as his own. In no way did he resemble the monster Dr. French had fabricated and brainwashed my sister into accepting.

Mom took a train back to Syracuse. In the station she met Alice, who actually did hand Eddie over to her. Alice kept her promise to stay in touch, but she never attempted to regain custody, though no legal transaction had transpired to prevent her from doing so.

Few people know the severe financial hardships through which our family struggled the next several years. And Eddie never overcame the insecurity of abandonment which resulted from his transfer between households at around two years of age. Mother admits he was the most difficult of all her children to raise. Eddie himself confesses to putting most of the gray hairs on Dad's head. In spite of the hardships, no one of us ever suggested we made a bad choice when Dad sent Mom to "go get our boy."

Six months after Eddie's return to us and fifteen years after Mother's most recent childbirth, Terry Lee arrived, undisputably Mom and Dad's "grand finale."

The son of his father's old age, Terry knew Daddy as we other children could never know him, for Terry had the unique privilege of being an only child after the rest of us had left home and were on our own.

One time while Daddy was making pastoral calls, he gave up trying to find a certain address. Leaving Terry in the car, Dad went to a nearby residence to ask directions. Terry watched as the woman of the house talked and gestured and talked some more. Dad finally returned to the car more confused than ever. Fumbling with the ignition, Terry heard Dad mutter, "Now I know how Balaam must have felt."

Dad often made Biblical references and applications but that one seemed vague and irrelevant to Terry until with a jolt it hit him! Dad, who never used expletives and rarely resorted to name calling, had effectively labeled that woman a lowly beast of burden.[2] But no hearer unfamiliar with Scripture would have been any wiser!

One final story completes this characterization of my dad. Early in this chapter, I told of the church my father pastored near Alva, Oklahoma where he not only established a congregation, but he helped the men of the congregation construct the original building on the present site.

Years later the congregation of that church celebrated their sixty-fifth anniversary by adding a steeple onto their building. The people reached into their past and named the new structure in honor of their first resident pastor, John E. McGraw. Rather than leaving his pastorates in disgrace, as Dr. French had implied to me, Dad left in such high regard that more than half a century later a congregation chose to honor him by dedicating their new addition in memory of his ministry among them.

The Man I Call Daddy!

In stark contrast, for a number of years a building at a well-respected theological institution wore Dr. French's name emblazoned across its face in bold letters. But you won't find his name there today, for those letters were hurriedly ripped off after the character of the man and the nature of his therapy were revealed to a stunned world and an embarrassed administration.

The identification of the man here portrayed is of utmost importance to me, for my own self-knowledge originates here. If what I know about my father, my mother and my family is not real, then I am without identity. If I do not know who they are, I do not know who I am, for they comprised the world into which I came and in which I grew up. If my father is not the man I have portrayed him to be, then I must conclude I am of unsound mind and never have known a sane moment.

University of Washington's adjunct professor of law, Elizabeth Loftus, a forensic psychologist and memory specialist who testifies in courts of law as an expert witness before numerous juries, expressed it this way:

> *How can you separate a man from his memory? If you take the memories away, haven't you also stripped him of his past, of all the precious, stored events that made him who he is? Without his memories, wouldn't [a man] fold up and die, an exterior scaffolding that has lost its inner structure and suddenly collapses in upon itself?*[3]

I believe this graphically describes what happened to my sister. Her memory obliterated by drugs, she found herself bereft of her real past, adrift without identity. She became a hollow exoskeleton, and as nature abhors a vacuum, her exterior scaffolding imploded. This, to me, explains her personality disintegration by the time she moved to the State of Washington, in desperate search of someone who would help her discover who she was and where she had come from.

By that time, an Oklahoma doctor had already set the direction for Lillian—a path of therapy-induced suggestion and blatant brainwashing, aided by use of hypnosis. In that environment a past was invented for her, giving to her a present identity and defining a role for her to play in the future.

She has embraced her role, accepting as fact the lie that she is the victim and survivor of incest. It is her prevailing focus. It consumes her and dictates much of what she is and what she does.

But if she is indeed the offspring of the man Dr. French described, and a victim of paternal incest, then the person that is me does not exist. As she told me so emphatically one day, "Donna, you can't have it both ways! You just can't have it both ways!"

On that we agree. Either our father was an all-too-rare example of a righteous man, or he was a pervert in cruel disguise. He was either a moral, loving parent, or he was an unconscionable pedophile, considered the lowest scum even in the pecking order within the walls of our prisons. He was a godly father, or a devilish predator. But he was not—could not be—both.

That delineates the chasm separating my sister Lillian and myself. She, too, derives her identity from her past. She is the sum of her memories, just as I am the totality of mine.

But one of us is dead wrong. One of us is a myth—deriving her identity from events that never happened and persons who never existed. One of us is a living, breathing lie.

One of us has no idea who she really is.

"You just can't have it both ways!"

CHAPTER NINE

Hanging Out the Dirty Laundry

My parents' time in Puerto Rico was drawing to a close. Expecting to stay three months, they spent two happy years on the island. At age seventy-four, Mother had impressed us all by learning enough Spanish to make herself understood.

As Mom was expanding her horizons, Dad's world was closing in on him. Alzheimer's disease was stealing his memories of the past and his hope of a future, while progressing deafness shut out much of his present. In the hope that more familiar surroundings would help decelerate his increasing confusion, arrangements were made for their return to the mainland.

Mother planned to visit all the children one more time before Dad required confinement. From Puerto Rico they planned to fly to Seattle, then to points south and east, finally to settle near my brother Peter's home in northwestern Oklahoma.

Peter was pastoring the same country church and living in the same parsonage that had been my parents' home for ten years. Now a comfortable mobile home awaited them just a few short steps from Peter's back door and across the yard from the old church building. Truly Mother and Dad were "coming home."

But for me, their homecoming constituted a crisis.

The summer of 1980, six months after I had heard Lillian's accusations of Dad, Lillian and her daughter Cheree had visited at our place in Terry, Montana for a few days. During her visit my sister continually spoke to me as if her accusations against Dad were established facts, ignoring my repudiation of them.

In particular I remember our conversation one afternoon as I hung laundry in the hot Montana sun. Lillian was speaking of the "incest," and she said with conviction, "I wish I could tell Mother."

With that statement, all the horror of my morning spent in Dr. French's office swept over me. I had been invited into that office precisely because Lillian had made an identical statement about me to Dr. French: "I wish I could tell Donna."

That night when I repeated Lillian's remark to my husband, his reaction echoed mine. As long as we had breath, Mother would never be subjected to what I had suffered, in spite of gag rules and resulting alienations if I broke them. Perhaps I underestimated Mom's strength, but I feared it would kill her.

Consequently, my folks' imminent return to the States and their plan to fly first to the Northwest indicated to me it was time to expose to my family Lillian's dirty little secret.

It was a sobering reality. To reveal charges made from within our own family against my father was sure to trigger a full-blown revolution. I had no way of knowing who would fight, who would retreat, or who would become a casualty. But I knew that no one near and dear to me would escape the carnage unscathed.

With much trepidation, I penned a letter to my sister Millie, warning her that as she made plans for the folks' flight home, she needed to know that Lillian had made serious accusations against Dad. For the life of me, I could not bring myself to write the word "incest."

That December marked my fortieth birthday. When Gary asked what I wanted to make this birthday special, I requested a phone call of unrestricted length to Millie in Santo Domingo.

Hanging Out the Dirty Laundry

Gary agreed, so Sunday afternoon I made my way to the phone in the Methodist Church in Chemung, Illinois, the place of our assignment at that time.

Only weeks shy of a full year since Lillian had disclosed her secret to me, I was surprised at how nervous I was making that phone call. As yet I had never had a conversation about this subject with a family member—other than my husband—who confirmed my belief that Lillian was dead wrong. Two sisters seemed to give her affirmation and support. Would this sister also take Lillian's side?

Dialing the phone number with unsteady hands, I stopped midway and hung up the receiver, not sure I had the courage to make this call after all. Sharing this information with Millie was going to be no easier than telling Gary. Once more I wavered between my own certainty that Dad was innocent and wondering how Lillian could make a false indictment with such conviction.

The sister next older than I, Millie was the one who often responded to my news items with a deflating, "I've known that for a long time. I just couldn't tell." Would that be her response now? Direct sometimes to the point of bluntness, she was not apt to dodge an issue or sugar-coat a response. I sat for some moments with my face in my hands, asking the Lord for strength to face whatever lay ahead.

I took the numbers slowly and carefully the next time. Nervous or not, I had to talk to Millie.

I need not have worried. While it was only with difficulty that I could use the word "incest", Millie harbored few inhibitions of any kind. When she had received my letter, she had read between the lines, remarking to her husband Bill, "There is only one thing so horrible that Donna wouldn't write it in a letter. Lillian has accused Daddy of incest."

Millie never graced the accusation with a flicker of credibility. I basked in the aura of her unwavering conviction, thinking, "This is more like it! This is how I expected every member of my family to respond." At that moment I judged Millie—my "craziest" sister— to be the most sane!

With relief I heard her say, "We could never send Mother into that situation unprepared. When we return to Puerto Rico for the Christmas holidays, I will tell her everything. If she still wants to fly to Seattle, she will go with full knowledge of what is happening there. I will instruct her that under no circumstance is she to go to Dr. French's office."

Millie was as clueless as I had been of the origin of Lillian's accusations, other than that they had been hatched in the head of her therapist. How he could successfully transplant them into Lillian's mind was beyond our comprehension.

Millie and I talked for an hour. For the first time in a year, I received from one of my sisters confirmation and support in my assessment of the situation. I was relieved and elated as I realized I no longer stood alone.

I also felt extremely sad. Mother bore the burden of watching Daddy slowly descend into the darkness of Alzheimer's disease. Now she would suffer the additional burden of knowing her husband had been falsely accused by a daughter. Could she hold up under such a heavy load? I even wondered if Mother would think I invented the whole story. After all, wasn't I as likely to be lying as Lillian?

In her usual no-nonsense manner, Millie had accepted the assignment of telling Mom about Lillian's accusations. Although Lillian's resentment and alienation were already known to Mother, the sordid details were sure to be a shock to her. To soften the blow, Millie first assured Mom of her own outrage and disbelief concerning Lillian's supposed memories.

Mother's response was predictably Mother. "Tell all the children of the charges and let them respond by revealing anything and everything they know."

Some have said Mom made a risky decision. I don't believe Mother considered it risky at all. She had no need to decide where truth resided, for she knew the truth. She had no twinge of doubt concerning Dad's character. She never for a moment feared that the other children, or anyone who really knew him, could confirm or believe such nonsense.

Mother weathered this storm as she had all the other challenges of her life. We don't know what inner battles she fought. Outwardly she modeled a woman anchored to the Rock, unruffled and confident. Even at her age, she personified the calm in the eye of the hurricane. Without so much as a discernable flinch, she remained fully confident in the Lord's provision, her husband's integrity, and in her children's collective ability to handle the situation appropriately.

As Mom requested, Millie and Bill prepared letters summarizing the situation, expressing all the outrage and disbelief the four of us felt at having our father and mother so implicated. They soundly denounced Dr. French—his character, his methods and his conclusions—as well as the actions of the daughters who had adopted his fantasies as their own realities.

With bated breath, we awaited the fallout from those not-so-subtle letters. We didn't have long to wait.

Many of Mother's children, learning of Lillian's charges for the first time, were stunned and furious at her claims. Some thought Millie and I had exaggerated her charges or that I had misunderstood and misconstrued Dr. French. Others had years ago observed behavior in Lillian that rendered her an unreliable source of information. Still others felt that I had no right to reveal to Millie what Lillian had confided to me, nor should Millie have blabbed it to the whole family.

Charges of betrayal abounded. Donna had betrayed Lillian. Lillian had betrayed Dad. Millie had betrayed Donna. Both Millie and I were denounced as responsible for an almost certain suicide attempt by Lillian. (We later learned that her husband intercepted the letters before she saw them.) Mother received phone calls assuring her that Dr. French was a capable and reliable therapist who was bringing restoration to Lillian; and that amateurs (specifically referring to Millie and me) should not be permitted to interfere.

Reactions and responses covered the spectrum, but one fact remained constant throughout the exchange. No hint of suspicion of any kind surfaced accusing Dad of abusing a child. Nor was any other offense attributed to either parent. We children might fault and condemn each other for creating family mayhem, but the characters and conduct of both Mother and Daddy emerged unassailed and unassailable by anyone other than Dr. French and those whose minds had been contaminated by him.

CHAPTER TEN

"Her Children . . . Call Her Blessed"

Born July 28, 1908, the first of two daughters to Clifton L. and Ida Willy Cummings, Opal Pauline found home to be a dugout, a dwelling literally carved out of a hillside in north central Oklahoma. The walls on three sides consisted of the dirt of the hill overlaid with boards. Mother described it as a "box with a lid."

When Opal entered first grade near Alva, each morning her father lifted her onto the back of the old work horse, then walked around to the animal's face, pointed toward the little schoolhouse three miles away and commanded, "School." Off the horse would go with Opal on board. When she arrived at school, the teacher helped her down and put the horse to graze. After school, the teacher placed her back on the horse and instructed the animal, "Home." And home they went.

During her high school years in Enid, earning her spending money by babysitting for friends and acquaintances, Opal discovered her greatest joy came from caring for children. She envisioned herself some day becoming the matron of an orphanage.

Skeletons Without Bones

Opal participated in the activities of the local church where her father served as Sunday school superintendent and classroom teacher. When the young people attended a rally at a church called Wesleyan Chapel, Opal and her friend Ruth (Nichols) Sanchez arrived early at the still-darkened building.

Soon the pastor, a single young man named John McGraw, began to light the kerosene lamps hanging along both outside walls. Taking note of the young man's agenda, the girls quickly developed one of their own.

A single center aisle led from the church's entrance to the platform. Pews on both sides of the aisle ran all the way to the outside walls. As John stepped between the pews and made his way to the outer wall, intent on lighting the lamp mounted above, the girls quickly seated themselves in that same pew.

When the pastor turned to retrace his steps, he found his progress blocked by two prim little maids waiting for the service to begin. Rather than crowd awkwardly past the girls, he took a giant stride over the pew in front of them and made his way to the young ladies, shaking their hands and welcoming them in the manner of all good pastors since time immemorial.

Returning to his task of lighting the lamps, John walked along another pew and put his match to the wick. Turning around, he once again found his way blocked by two young women who had decided this pew was more to their liking than the last. John grinned good naturedly, nodded a greeting, and once again swung his long limbs over the back of the pew just ahead.

Little did that pastor know that some eight years later one of those capricious teenagers would become his bride.

After attending Miltonvale Wesleyan College in Kansas, Opal returned to Enid, joining Pastor Paul and Olive Hodge in a musical ministry. Opal also helped care for their young children.

While Opal was living in the Hodge home, Olive reported to her that Pastor John McGraw, recently widowed, had asked if he might call on Opal. Opal responded without enthusiasm. But John persisted and Opal, acting on Mrs. Hodges' advice, accepted his invitation, intending to tell him that she was not interested in his attentions.

When the date actually transpired, Opal somehow forgot all about her carefully prepared speech.

But John didn't forget his. He told her he wanted her to become his wife! Ten months later on May 5, 1933, Pastor Hodge united John McGraw and Opal Cummings in marriage at the Enid Wesleyan Church. Someone remarked to Mother that it was the skinniest wedding ever celebrated in that church!

The honeymoon trip, witnessed by well-wishers, consisted of Dad pushing Mom around the town square in a baby buggy in an old-fashioned shivaree. He must have impressed Mom with his ability to maneuver the vehicle; she kept him pushing baby buggies for the next twenty-five years!

The Great Depression gripped the nation, while "dust bowl" conditions scourged its mid-section. The parched dirt was not only underfoot, but dry winds kept much of it aloft, filling eyes, noses and lungs of man and beast alike. It felt like grit between your teeth, sandpaper in your hair and gravel in your shoes. Sheets and blankets dipped in water and hung over doors and windows filtered out some of the dust before it landed on food, furniture and floors.

Over the next ten years Dad pastored churches throughout Oklahoma and Texas, and Mother gave birth to four daughters and one son.

In 1943 an opportunity arose for Dad to work in the publishing department of our church headquarters located "back east." Dad called together the church and college leaders he most respected. In prayer they sought to discover God's will regarding Dad's employment opportunity.

Confident that God was leading, Dad went on ahead to find housing and begin his new job. As Mother waited for the end of the school year, she packed our belongings and arranged for the moving of our household possessions.

What excitement to travel all the way to New York State by rail! World War II filled trains with military personnel. Unable to

Skeletons Without Bones

sit together, we felt fortunate to all have seats in the same railroad car. When the conductor came to punch our tickets, Mother held up her eight, and pointing, she said, "These are for this one, and that one, and there's one over there...." One conductor responded, "Are all these children *yours*?" Mother retorted, "You don't think I'd be taking someone else's kids on a trip like this, do you?"

Meals purchased on board were beyond our means. When the other passengers made their way to the dining car, we gathered in the vacated seats around Mother. She pulled out a huge black suitcase filled with non-perishables. We devoured our crackers and cheese and peanut butter, and scrambled back to our seats before the return of the dining car patrons.

At Chicago, Mother assigned suitcases and packages to each of us, put big kids in charge of little kids, and herded us all off the train. She found a driver to take our unlikely entourage to the second depot where we would embark on the final leg of our journey. Mother counted us, instructed us, checked for forgotten packages and opened her purse expecting to pay our fare. The driver intervened.

"Lady, anyone traveling across the country with that many children doesn't owe me a thing." With that, he was gone.

Somehow Mother managed to get us all to Syracuse before the black suitcase was totally empty. Dad had purchased a big house on Sunnycrest Road and we were ready to fill it.

But not for long. A church in nearby Baldwinsville asked Dad to fill its pulpit in the absence of a resident pastor. For some months the whole mob of us made the thirty-mile trip by bus each Sunday morning and returned to Syracuse by bus that same evening.

When temporary pastor became permanent pastor, our house went up for rent and we moved to Baldwinsville.

Originally built as a single-family dwelling, the church building's lower floor had been converted into a sanctuary and the upstairs became residence for the pastor's family. The contractor could not have foreseen a parsonage family as large as ours. Now the bus trips changed direction as Dad commuted to Syracuse to work each week day.

World War II raged on. I vaguely remember the rationing of food, particularly sugar. Each of us had a card with our name on it. The corner grocer tracked purchases by punching holes in the cards. You felt proud when it was your card that provided sugar for the whole family that week. Mother calculated each rationed item, stretching it until the next cards were received.

Who could forget the eerie blackouts? When the air raid sirens wailed, all lights were extinguished until the "all clear" signal sounded.

We discovered how strictly the "all lights out" rule was enforced. During one drill, a knock sounded on our door. Even Dad was too cautious to open the door to an unidentified visitor in the pitch darkness of an air raid! But it proved to be a most unhappy officer who had detected a single light bulb burning in our basement, in spite of the cardboard carefully nailed over the windows. We all listened as he lectured that even a pinpoint of light provided a target for enemy aircraft. He did not feel that one woman's need to do the family laundry warranted risking a national calamity!

The combined incomes from Dad's pastorate and his Syracuse job scarcely covered the expenses of our large household. Mother decided to help make up the difference by becoming a foster parent. After all, caring for children was what she loved to do.

When we were duly certified by the New York State Welfare Department, they brought us a three-month-old boy. Mother took one look at him and said, "Oh, no, I can't take this child. I have my own children here to consider."

Mother thought the lethargic child had some terrible disease. His arms and legs were pencil thin, his belly was so distended he appeared to be deformed.

The welfare lady assured Mother the baby posed no threat to the health of the other children, but Mother remained unconvinced, agreeing the child could stay only until another home could be found.

Mother immediately took Roger to her trusted family doctor for his assessment. He diagnosed a severe case of malnutrition and sent Mother home with a prescribed formula. Mother understood now why Roger reminded her of the newspaper pictures of refugee children. He was literally starving, just as they were.

Babies needing nourishing food was one problem Mom knew how to handle. He was a pathetic sight, but if he posed no threat to the other children, Mom was ready to do battle with Roger's condition. Ignoring the doctor's store-bought formula, she got busy and whipped up some of her trusty oatmeal gruel.

When the welfare woman returned to remove the child Mother had said she couldn't keep, the astonished caseworker didn't recognize him! She actually said, "This is not the baby I brought you a week and a half ago." His arms and legs had filled out, his bloated belly had shrunk, and his big brown eyes sparkled.

Both ladies—Mother and the social worker—agreed it would be a mistake to remove the child, and Roger became a forever member of our family. It is no surprise it turned out that way, for I never knew a baby who, given a few days under Mom's care, didn't flourish. And I never knew Mother not to fall head-over-heels in love with every infant she took in her arms. The New York State Welfare took note of those two facts and did not hesitate to take advantage of them whenever it was in the best interest of one of their wards.

Caring for foster children was only one way Mother contributed to the family income. During the war, factories begged women to fill vacancies left by G.I.'s. Mother hired a babysitter and went to work in the Onondaga Pottery. Now both our parents made daily bus rides into Syracuse.

At the pottery Mother met a young woman named Katrina. Upon learning Katrina's last name, Mother asked, "Could you be related to my foster child who has the same last name as yours?" Bingo! Mom had just discovered Roger's birth mother.

Though the welfare refused to release information that would allow natural parents and foster parents to contact each other, they could not prevent a chance meeting such as this. Both of Roger's mothers welcomed the relationship. Katrina received frequent updates on her son while Mom learned something of Roger's history.

Later, when Katrina was strong enough to leave the sanitorium where she was convalescing, my folks became her sponsors and she joined our lively household for approximately two years. Then the welfare decided it was probably confusing for Roger to have two mothers in the same household, so Katrina took an apartment close enough to assure continued contact with her son.

I'm not sure how long Mother continued to work at the pottery. But one day while riding the bus to work, she felt impressed to go home. She tried to shake off the impression as a case of maternal jitters. But when the feeling persisted, she became convinced the Lord was trying to tell her something wasn't right at home. She made up her mind that as soon as she arrived at work, she would notify her boss that she needed to go home.

Her decision brought her no peace. The urgency persisted, and she finally concluded that God was insisting she should go home—not later, but *now*!

When the bus arrived downtown, she passed up the coach destined for the pottery and boarded one that made the return trip to Baldwinsville.

At home Mother found her three pre-schoolers alone, with no sign of the babysitter who had been there when Mom left for work. I was standing half way down the stairway leading to our second story apartment, crying hysterically. Lillian and Roger were upstairs, still in their beds.

We had no phone but an irate Mother marched next door and dialed a number. When the sitter picked up the receiver, Mother instructed the young woman not to return, ever. Mother did not need her services. Others would have to fill vacancies in factories. Mother had a job at home which she would never again trust to anyone else.

Those were indeed momentous times. The adults would huddle around the radio which stood in our living room, an impressive piece of furniture the size of a bookcase. Daddy splurged on that bit of affluence in order to track world events.

I was too young to comprehend much of what was going on, but when Japan surrendered, I knew the horror of war had ended and that we had won! I don't know how the rest of the world celebrated but I remember what happened in our small corner.

Mother supervised and supplied the raw materials as my sister Millie designed hats for us kids out of oatmeal box lids. They were painted red, white, and blue, and threaded with yarn to tie under our chins. The cylindrical boxes, tied around our necks, became drums. Mother donated some of her pots and pans for even louder drums and cymbals. Lining us up parade fashion, Millie marched us all around our block, celebrating victory. For once in our lives, we made all the noise we could muster and the adults we met responded in kind!

Mother had quit her job to be home with her children, but she did more than take care of us kids. She was Sunday school superintendent, Sunday school teacher and church pianist. She also visited the sick and shut-ins. When one of my classmates contracted polio, Mother took me to see her. That was my first encounter with a monster known as an iron lung. It hissed and wheezed and occasionally sighed while I stood at her shoulder and visited with Margaret's image in the mirror propped in front of her. Meanwhile, Mom comforted and prayed with the over-wrought mother.

Before long the Welfare Department had another child for Mother. The same age as my older brother, this ten-year-old had been in every imaginable kind of trouble. If Mother could not salvage him, he would be sent to reform school.

The experiment was doomed before Mom had a chance. The boy lied about everything. He went to church long enough to find out where they put the offering baskets, then he stole the money collected to purchase Sunday school supplies.

He didn't stay long. Mother dared not risk having him around her children or the children of the church families. After that she accepted only babies and toddlers from the Welfare Office.

Dad pastored that little church known as "Beacon Gospel Tabernacle" in Baldwinsville for four years, after which we returned to Syracuse. My growing up years from fourth grade through my junior year in high school were spent in our house on Sunnycrest Road.

"Her Children . . . Call Her Blessed"

Mother continued to keep foster children, most of whom needed temporary placement while their families were in crisis. Sometimes, though, the case worker called to say they needed a permanent home for a child "that would just fit into your family."

Marie was ten months old when the ill health of her first foster mother required the child's placement in another home.

Soon after her arrival, Mother stumbled onto Marie's roots. Once a week after school Mother would hostess a neighborhood Bible Club in our home. Erla Flanagan, working with an organization called *Child Evangelism*, would set up her flannelgraph board and prepare for the impending influx of neighborhood children.

When Miss Flanagan met Marie, she said, "Why, I know this little girl. She is from another home in which I have been conducting a Bible Club."

Armed with name and phone number, Mother contacted the Buchanans, Marie's former family. After Mrs. Buchanan's surgery, Mother arranged the first of several visits of their entire family to our home.

When Marie graduated from her crib, she became resident little sister in the single bed opposite the double bed occupied by Lillian and me.

Marie proved to be a special addition to our family. The youngest girl and surrounded in the family line-up by boys, she and Mother formed an exceptional relationship that continues to this day.

In our house an empty crib proved too much for Mother to endure and more than the Welfare could ignore. When they called with yet another child, Mother reminded them, "But I already have more children than you allow. Our bedrooms are all full."

To no one's surprise, the crib soon was occupied by a curly-headed little bundle of energy named John. As handsome as he was good-natured, John bubbled his way into our hearts. His birth mother was confined to a hospital and the father had several older children to care for. Unwilling to relinquish his son to the finality of adoption, he allowed John to be placed in a foster home.

The crib's next occupant was our darling Jeanette, who forever remains a baby in our minds, for we never saw her grow up. Eight months later Eddie came charging into our lives, in every way the total antithesis of Jeanette but every bit as lovable.

Keeping welfare children allowed Mother to contribute to the family income while she did what she most enjoyed. Mom loved us all equally, giving extra time and attention to whichever child needed it most. She didn't make distinctions between us because of our origins. Once when Roger "mouthed off" to Mom in typical teenage fashion, I jumped in with both feet, railing at him about how grateful he should be that Mother and Dad gave him a home and declaring he had no right to speak to Mother in such a manner. Mom quietly squelched my tirade by saying pointedly, "Donna, Roger has all the same rights that you have."

However, there were times when of necessity we were delineated into categories, in spite of what Mother may have preferred.

The Welfare Department supplied each foster child with a generous allowance for clothing. We non-welfare kids looked on with envy every fall and spring as one by one Mother took the foster children to town and outfitted them with new clothes from head to toe.

While "we" got along with hand-me-downs and make-overs, "they" were quite resplendent in new items we never dreamed of owning. They had winter coats, spring coats, rain coats, school coats, play coats, dress coats, and even house coats! They could get Sunday shoes, play shoes, school shoes, tennis shoes, snow boots and rain boots, and real slippers!

Sometimes Mother would come home from a shopping trip fuming and fussing because she had seen other families outfitting their foster children. In the process, items of clothing for their "not foster" children would be purchased with the unwary state picking up the tab.

Mother was too honest for such opportunism. We would go without new clothes before she would stretch the welfare clothing allowance to include a single item for one of her non-welfare children.

"Her Children . . . Call Her Blessed"

It is impossible for me to comprehend how Mother managed those tumultuous years in Syracuse. Living under one roof she had children who were working full time jobs, children who were students in college, high school, junior high and grade school, as well as pre-schoolers and babies. In addition, married children and grandchildren would come home during holidays and summer vacations. The basement bulged with young men who boarded with us, and Roger's mother lived with us as she made her way to personal independence. Add to that an assortment of playmates and best friends, and at any given moment you could find kids upstairs, kids downstairs, kids in the basement, kids in the attic, kids on the porches and kids in the yard. Often there were kids in the trees.

Shortage of finances was always a problem. On her limited budget, Mom navigated and orchestrated the family through weddings, holidays, graduations, measles, school schedules, broken appliances, church events and weather extremes. She remained unruffled as she prayed her teenagers through budding romances, broken romances, lack of romances, and much-too-intense or hanging-on-too-long romances.

She shopped, cooked, cleaned, did laundry and tracked kids. But often we used up at a quicker pace than she could replace, devoured more than she could prepare, dirtied more rapidly than she could clean and cluttered faster than she could pick up. We filled clothes hampers quicker than she could fill a washing machine. Some of us kept soiled bed linen an on-going challenge. And tracking that many kids would have kept a full-blown police department in a panic.

Mother managed it all with a serene spirit. Sometimes chaos reigned, the house resembled a disaster zone, the laundry pile dwarfed Pike's Peak and dirty dishes grew to the size of rickety skyscrapers. After all, kids—even when they travel in packs—are well able to melt into the woodwork when there is work to be done. But Mother remained unharried and unhurried.

In fact, we children often teased that if she moved any slower, she would be going backwards. In retrospect, I think Mom had figured out that she didn't have to move at all to keep up with her kids. As life whirled about her, she was the eye in the middle of the tornado, the calm in the midst of the hurricane. From that vantage point, she could reach out and touch all the action without moving with it and without being moved by it.

Though she functioned in one gear and that gear was "slow," Mom was not a passive spectator. She was in charge of that bustling household, even in its wildest moments, but she was not consumed by it. By all appearances, she thrived on it. To top it all, one year she along with Dad enrolled in night classes at our high school and together they learned to type.

No doubt we would have remained New Yorkers indefinitely had not a fire devoured our church headquarters building where Dad and my brother Peter were employed.

It seemed as if Indiana were the other side of the world. Mother faced the distinct possibility of losing her four foster children, and in fact did lose one of them for the better part of a year. Peter was engaged to be married, and rather than leave his bride-to-be, she was included in our trek west. Millie graduated from college that spring and returned home in time to move to Indiana with us.

Moving from a large eastern city to a small, midwestern town caused a fair amount of culture shock. Not to any of us—we had no culture to shock. I fear it was easier for us to adapt to small-town ways than for the small town to adjust to us. But the resilient community managed to make a remarkable recovery as it absorbed the jolt occasioned by the invading horde that swarmed in, out and around the house on Adams Street near the high school.

They welcomed us with midwest hospitality. With the mother of the clan at age forty-nine beginning to show an expanding waistline, she could scarcely go anywhere without being showered with solicitous questions and courteous attentions. Mom was embarrassed by it all, especially when men asked how she was feeling. Her last pregnancy had been fifteen years before. "Back then men didn't ask those kinds of questions of a woman in my condition."

But Mom took it in stride, saying, "If I'm going to have a baby like a young woman, I'd better learn to take the attention like a young woman."

"Her Children . . . Call Her Blessed"

Even after Peter and his fiancee married and became a separate household, money remained an elusive commodity. Sometimes it seemed non-existent. When the washing machine quit working, Mother knew the cost was twenty-five dollars to replace the broken belt—twenty-five dollars more than she had.

Laundry became a formidable foe as it grew exponentially with each passing day. Finding clean clothes became a crisis rivalled by discovering places to put dirty ones. Mother endured it until it reached critical mass, then she gathered a virtual mountain range of dirty clothes and sorted it into more manageable foothills around the kitchen floor. She loaded the defunct washer and added detergent, all the while talking to her heavenly Father.

"Now you know, Lord, I can't send children to school in dirty clothes. I can't leave babies unchanged. When you were on earth you fixed broken bodies. Now I need you to fix the broken belt on this washing machine." Whereupon she set the dial and turned it on.

And it worked! It churned its agitator in the manner of all good washers. Eddie, our ever-inquisitive toddler, came into the kitchen to assess the situation.

"Mom, did somebody come fix the washing machine?"

"Yes, Eddie, Somebody fixed the washing machine."

"But no one came. I didn't see anybody come."

"You know I didn't have any money to have someone come fix it, Eddie. So I asked Jesus to fix it and He did."

Eddie started looking behind doors and in all the nooks and crannies, saying, "But I didn't get to see Him. Where did He go after He fixed the washer? I want to see Him."

That washing machine continued to do our laundry for a complete year, after which it expired, worn beyond repair. This time the problem was solved in a more orthodox but less dramatic fashion—Dad bought a new one. Considering our financial situation, that may have been the greater miracle!

We children grew up knowing that though Mother and Dad had limited resources, they were on good terms with the One who knew no such limitations. They had no gimmicks, no formulas, no magic tricks. Just a simple faith that said, "I've done all I can do, Lord. Now I need You to do what You can do." Then they rested in the knowledge that "all things work together for good to them that love God, to them who are the called according to his purpose" (Romans 8:28 KJV).

Mother was the disciplinarian of the family. Meting out punishment was Dad's one malleable area, and we children were shameless to take advantage of it. Doubtless Mom's no-nonsense approach to retribution was designed to counterbalance Dad's ambivalent one. Her philosophy was simple and straightforward. She doled out a ready supply of love, garnished as needed with spankings that were designed to not need repeating.

As her name Opal indicates, Mom is a jewel, a mother among mothers who raised eleven children who "rise up and call her blessed."

Mom's years are numbered now. My hope is that Lillian, the only dissenting voice among Mother's children, will soon be able to discard the falsehoods she has accumulated over these past two decades and discover her true inheritance, uncorrupted and uncorroded—pure gold ready for the taking. For truly, Mother deserves to know in this lifetime, as well as in the next, that *all* her children call her blessed.

CHAPTER ELEVEN

Documenting the Past

Two months of meetings in Upstate New York in 1980 provided for me an ideal opportunity to reconstruct events of my childhood.

One of our first engagements that spring was at the Wesleyan Church of Sandy Creek, not far from Lake Ontario. As we entered the town, a sign invited travelers to visit the local Methodist Church, giving the pastor's name as Rev. Ivan Greenfield.

I was stunned to see what could only be the fingerprint of the Almighty upon the task I had undertaken. Thirty years before, a young man with that name had attended our church in Baldwinsville and had come under my father's tutelage. He had become a close friend to our family and had married a young lady from our church. Later he had become a Methodist minister. It seemed unlikely that two ministers named Ivan Greenfield would simultaneously pastor Methodist churches in Upstate New York!

Rev. Greenfield came to the Saturday night service looking much as I remembered him from my childhood. After Gary and I had

Skeletons Without Bones

sung a couple of songs, Ivan stood and with tears flowing down his cheeks, he spoke of my father's godly influence upon him as a young man. He told of his own call to the ministry and how under Dad's counsel he had attended Houghton College for his ministerial training.

Witnessing to my dad's imprint on his young life, Ivan unknowingly referenced the very time and place described to me in Lillian's letter accusing Dad of molesting her. "The room behind the platform" was located in the church Ivan mentioned, the same church Dr. French insisted Dad had been forced to leave in disgrace. Rev. Greenfield would never know what it meant to me to hear him accurately describe those real events and actual situations. "Thank you, Lord, for leaving your fingerprints for me to see."

My encounter with Rev. Greenfield was totally uncontrived, but we deliberately sought out other individuals and places in New York State. Gary and I visited that little mission in Baldwinsville that had been our home in my early years. Situated one block from the old Erie Canal, it now looked old and run down to me.

In a nursing home in that same town we found Eva Greene, a dear friend of my parents, now nearly one hundred years old. Mrs. Greene's mind was amazingly sharp and she gladly reminisced about my parents' ministry there. She recalled how after we had moved away from Baldwinsville, she had asked Dad if he would drive from Syracuse once a week to hold a Bible study in her home. Dad conducted that Bible study for a number of years, later adding a Sunday evening service. Often one or more of us children accompanied our parents to those meetings held in our former hometown.

When that Bible study grew too large for Mrs. Greene's living room, Dad spoke to the officials of the Wesleyan Conference about establishing a church in the growing town of Baldwinsville. Before we left town that day, Gary and I drove out to view the beautiful church that had resulted from that little Bible study/prayer group Daddy had nurtured years before.

So Dr. French's alleged pedophile had indeed left a trail—not the sordid one he had intimated, but an honored and respected one that belied Dr. French's warped conclusions.

Next Gary and I drove to Syracuse where our experiences followed a similar pattern. Every evening service brought additional witnesses who verified the high esteem held for my parents. I tried not to show an undue interest in their comments, but inwardly I basked in the sunshine of their disclosures.

Some people drove substantial distances just to visit and pay homage to my parents who had played an important role in their lives. They recalled real memories that made sense to me, not false ones dredged up from some therapist's cranial cesspools.

One other significant encounter took place in south central New York. Rev. I. Leslie Conley and his wife Faye attended a service we held in Elmira. My folks had known the Conleys in Oklahoma before my birth. Later Rev. Conley had been our pastor in New York State when we moved from Baldwinsville back to Syracuse. Their only daughter Joy had been Lillian's best friend all through elementary school.

Visiting with the Conleys, they spoke of our little "Sunbeam Quartet" that consisted of Joy and Lillian, our friend Marjorie and me. Mrs. Conley had accompanied us on the piano and served as our coach and director.

The Conleys immediately asked about Lillian. I hedged a little by telling them I had seen her only rarely in the last several years. Then without revealing my real intent, I asked them what they remembered most about Lillian.

Mrs. Conley laughed at my request and said without hesitation, "I remember Lillian always wanted to play doctor. We bought Joy a little nurse's kit. It was the game Lillian most often wanted to play, only she would not be the nurse. Joy had to be the nurse, because Lillian always had to be the doctor."

In Dr. French's office I had been told that my father had put it into Lillian's head that she *had* to become a doctor. But Faye Conley, without prompting, substantiated that as a very young child, Lillian already showed interest in being a doctor. Even that early, Lillian had spoken of her dream to someday become a missionary doctor like Dr. Marilyn Birch. I remember it clearly because, although I was two years her senior, I had no clear idea of what I wanted to be. Certainly I had no such lofty ambitions, which I felt must indicate a deficiency in my character. I often envied Lillian's fixed and unwavering goal which kept her focused during her high school years and influenced her selection of college courses.

It is natural that Dad would have supported and encouraged Lillian in her dream, but to make it his rapacious ambition for his daughter constituted pure maniacal nonsense.

Later, when I told the Conleys of Lillian's accusations of Daddy, they reacted with the same shock and disbelief as the Scotts had displayed. They, too, refuted everything that had been told to me in Dr. French's office. They had known Lillian as a normal, happy, friendly child, displaying none of the aberrant characteristics and behaviors that Dr. French and Lillian had ascribed to her. The Lillian they knew was a little girl without fears of her father or misgivings toward her home. They authenticated there were no unpublished reasons why Dad had changed churches. They assured me, "If there had been, we would have been privy to that information. Furthermore, if the officials had reason to remove him from pastorates, they would not have employed him in their International Headquarters until he reached retirement age, nor would they have sent him back into the pastorate for ten more years after his retirement."

Once again I had to wonder at French's complete disinterest in checking his theories and his disregard for readily obtainable facts. I had, in fact, sent him the names, addresses and phone numbers of the persons in authority over Dad, and asked him to investigate for himself.[1]

Family friends were not my only source of information during those years of our traveling ministry. At every opportunity we visited all the relatives we could impose upon. In that way, one by one I learned how each person felt about the accusations leveled by Lillian and about the disclosure I had made a year later concerning her accusations.

To my surprise, I discovered that Dad had not been the only family member implicated by Lillian to have been guilty of making unwelcome sexual overtures toward her. Thankfully, these additional accusations were later retracted by Lillian as being untrue. But damage had been done and the original stories had spread too far for the retractions to ever catch up.

Statistics show this to be the typical pattern of false accusations of sexual abuse. The memories take on a life of their own, an unseen monster devouring relatives, friends and even strangers as it seeks to assuage its voracious appetite for more victims and more bizarre incidents. After all, audiences dwindle when all the news is old news. Retaining the limelight requires new material and fresh audiences.

As information was compared, bits and pieces heretofore individually known but unshared, there emerged a composite picture of Lillian's young adulthood that had gone undetected. Some accounts came from brothers and sisters with whom Lillian had lived during her coming-to-adulthood years. Others came from brothers and sisters who had boarded with Lillian during their student years.

Signs had surfaced way back there that Lillian had found it difficult to recognize and deal with her real world. She no doubt found herself overloaded and overwhelmed as she took difficult pre-med college courses. To meet college expenses, she worked long hours in hospitals or taught high school subjects in hard-to-manage, inner-city classrooms. In addition, she married and gave birth to a daughter.

Meanwhile, she reportedly lived mostly on potato chips and pop, most likely falling back on her former crutches of uppers to propel her through the days and downers to sedate her through the nights.

The details I gathered came one fragment at a time. They were told to me reluctantly, and only after Lillian leveled her accusations against Dad. The consensus of those who were close to Lillian during her post high school years was that Lillian's own actions and behaviors had long ago destroyed her credibility with them. To their credit, they had kept their conclusions to themselves until they felt that Lillian herself had tipped their hands toward full disclosure.

However, had I personally been aware of these facts, I would have been less traumatized and better equipped to question Lillian's credibility in Dr. French's office.

Within the family, we still disagreed among ourselves whether Dr. French played the villain or the hero in all this. Whereas Lillian had once been self-destructive and reclusive—the worst case Dr. French had ever encountered—she was now emerging with coping and social skills, nothing short of a miracle wrought by Dr. French's wonderful patience and skillful handling. It is hard to discount success.

Even Mother, during a visit to me, suggested that I was too hard on Dr. French. "If Lillian is getting better, he must be doing something right. If Anna and Ginny consider him to be credible, surely he can't be all bad. Don't you think you could be mistaken?"

I knew Mother could not possibly know all we had discovered about him. Neither did I want her to know. But how could I convince her that Dr. French's "wisdom" was pure poison without hurting her further?

Knowing she liked to read, I handed her my volume of Janov's *Primal Scream*, and said, "Mother, this is the book Dr. French makes all his clients read. He adheres to and practices what it teaches. Read it and tell me what you think of it."

For the next day or two she waded through the putrid psychobabble of that volume. Three or four chapters into it, I figured she had doubtless had enough.

"How do you like that book, Mother? Do you still think I am too hard on Dr. French?"

She wrinkled her nose in a grimace as she replied, "I don't think you are nearly hard enough!"

CHAPTER TWELVE

Westward Ho!

The mid-eighties thrust major changes upon our lives. At eighty-four years of age, Daddy was promoted from nursing home to heavenly home. Sorrow mingled with relief as we celebrated his escape from the constraints of failing mind and body. Lillian did not join us as we put Dad to rest, and I was glad she chose not to come. Immersed in *real* memories, I had neither appetite nor energy to contend with her false ones.

That same year our son Dustin left the nest, bound for college. Soon after, we "left the road," ending twenty-two years of itinerant ministry. As our boys reached adolescence, it appeared our style of musical ministry had reached obsolescence. Ironically, we found ourselves retiring our motor home and looking for careers whereas our peers were retiring from careers and looking for motor homes.

The changes were coming too fast for comfort. Gary's hometown of Terry, Montana, where we made our home, yielded few employment opportunities. Abandoned real estate and business establishments deteriorated while the Census Bureau projected even greater population loss during the next decade.

Hope blossomed anew as we accepted an invitation to help "grow" a church in Arizona. But the blossom withered quickly and the move proved to be a disaster for us. Faced with the prospect of returning to the familiar hopelessness of eastern Montana, I suffered a complete breakdown which required a two-year recovery time.

A glimmer of light appeared on the western horizon when Ginny and Lyle encouraged us to move to Washington State where carpentry and clerical opportunities abounded. They even offered us a landing place in their big house, thus delaying for them an empty nest as their youngest left for college.

So it was in August of 1989 following our son Dustin's wedding in Roundup, Montana, Ginny and Lyle had a passenger on board when they returned to Western Washington. We were still skittish from our Arizona debacle, so Gary and Shane remained in Montana while I went to "spy out the land." A few days later I called to tell Gary to start packing. Within the month, we closed down our place in Montana and arrived bag and baggage to take advantage of Ginny and Lyle's offer before they could reconsider. As Ginny had predicted, Gary quickly found employment doing carpentry work and I landed a clerical job.

During the year we lived with Ginny, her daughters and sons-in-law took their turns going through Dr. French's "intensive therapy." They also regularly attended a Bible study conducted by French, and Lillian continued to see him weekly, although she declared herself well and no longer in need of therapy.

Following years of estrangement, Lillian and I had gradually developed a better relationship. Chatting on the phone and doing things together, we avoided any reference to our different pasts. I could not tell whether her acceptance of me stemmed from her personal desire to make peace, or whether she wanted to prove herself well enough to forgive my sin against her. To other family members she still spoke with some heat regarding my "betrayal" of her, but she never exhibited to me any remaining animosity.

By fall of 1990, established in permanent positions, Gary and I, with our younger son Shane, moved from Ginny and Lyle's house into our own home.

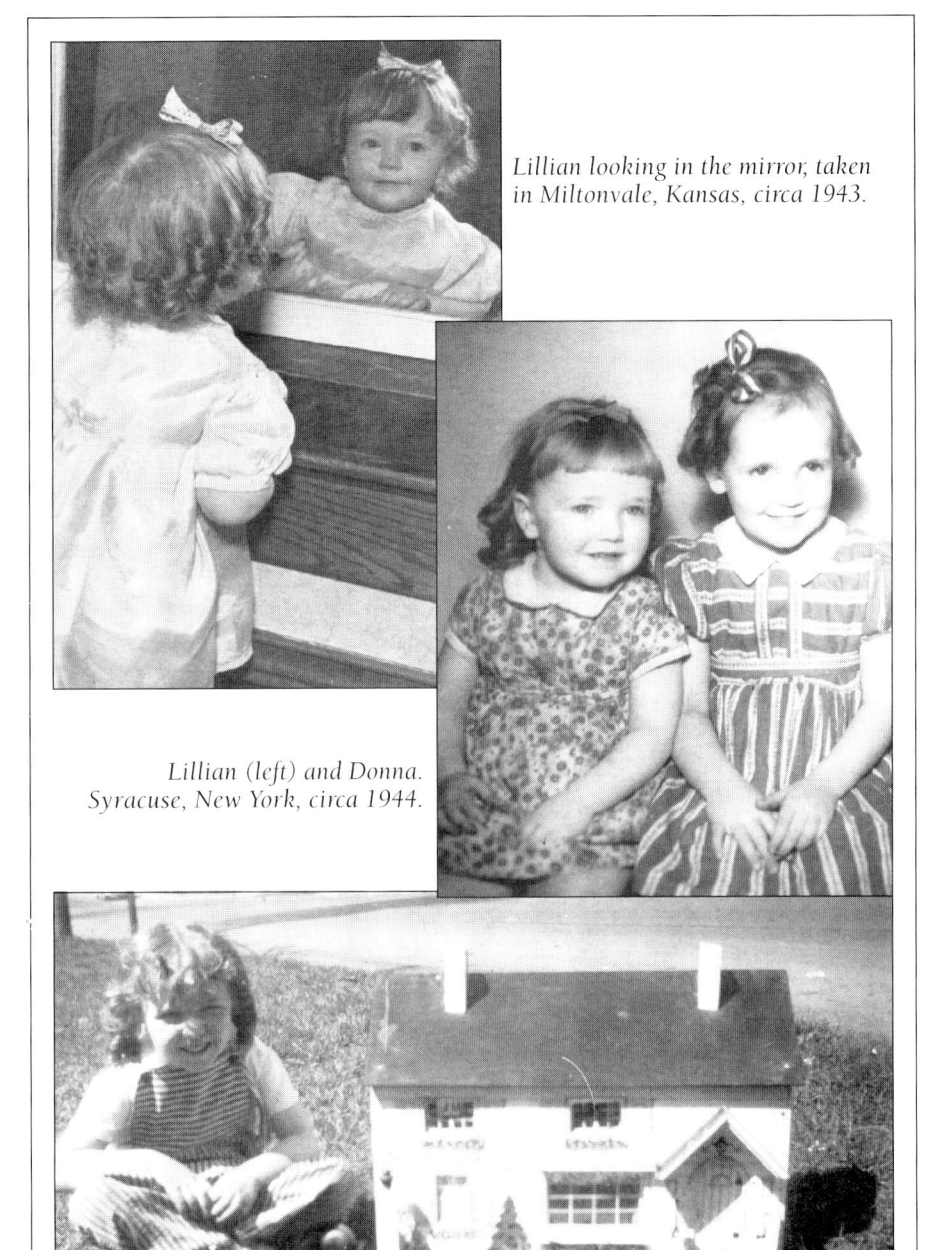

Lillian looking in the mirror, taken in Miltonvale, Kansas, circa 1943.

Lillian (left) and Donna. Syracuse, New York, circa 1944.

Lillian beside our doll house.

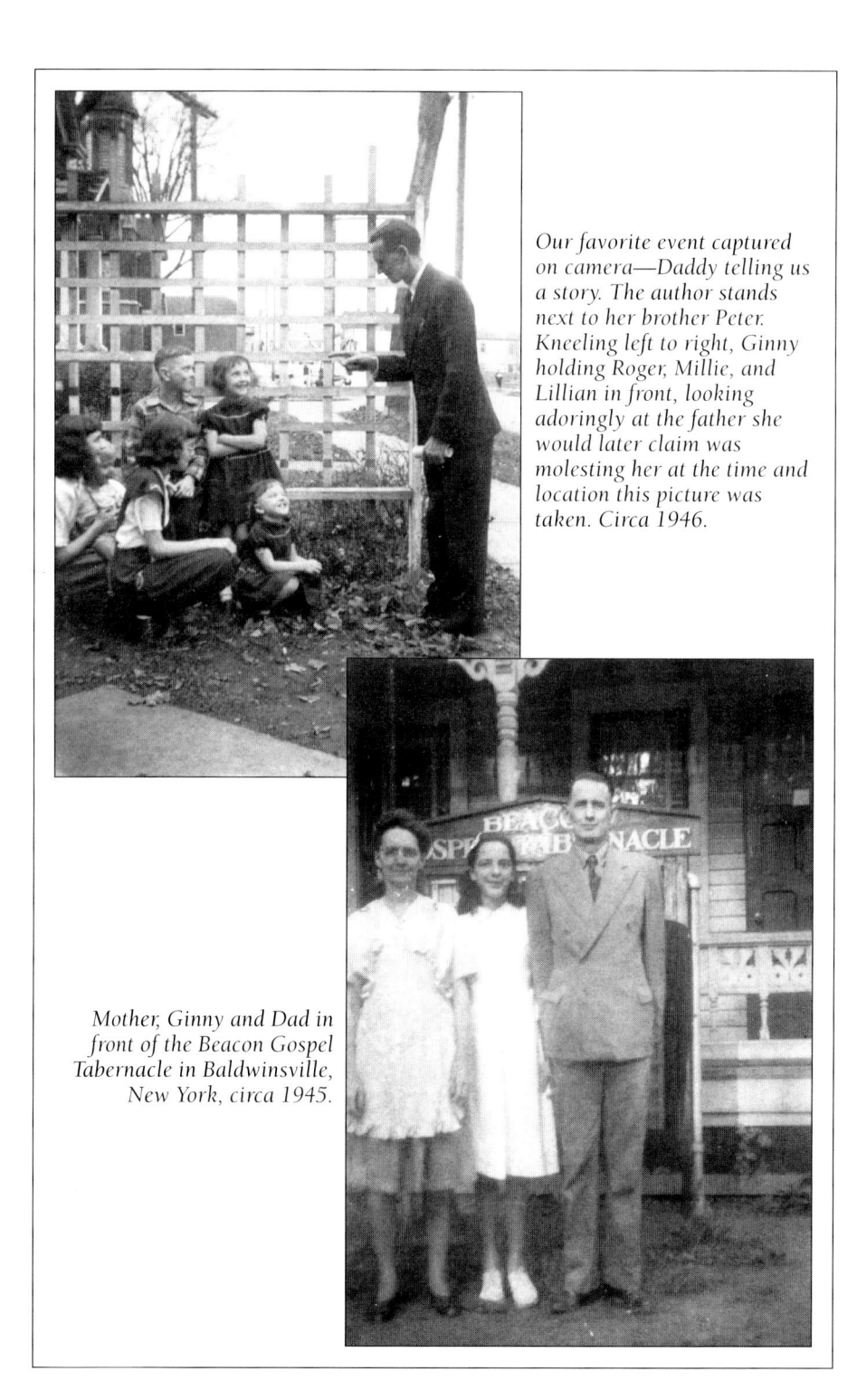

Our favorite event captured on camera—Daddy telling us a story. The author stands next to her brother Peter. Kneeling left to right, Ginny holding Roger, Millie, and Lillian in front, looking adoringly at the father she would later claim was molesting her at the time and location this picture was taken. Circa 1946.

Mother, Ginny and Dad in front of the Beacon Gospel Tabernacle in Baldwinsville, New York, circa 1945.

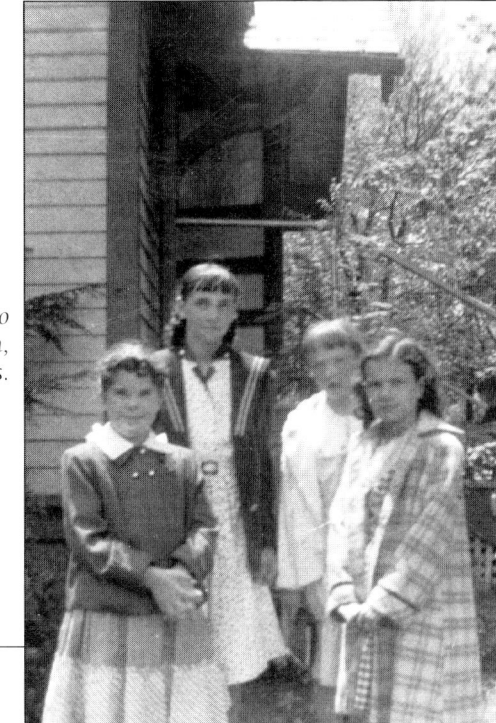

The Sunbeam Quartet, left to right: Joy Conley, Donna, Lillian, and Marjorie Bajus.

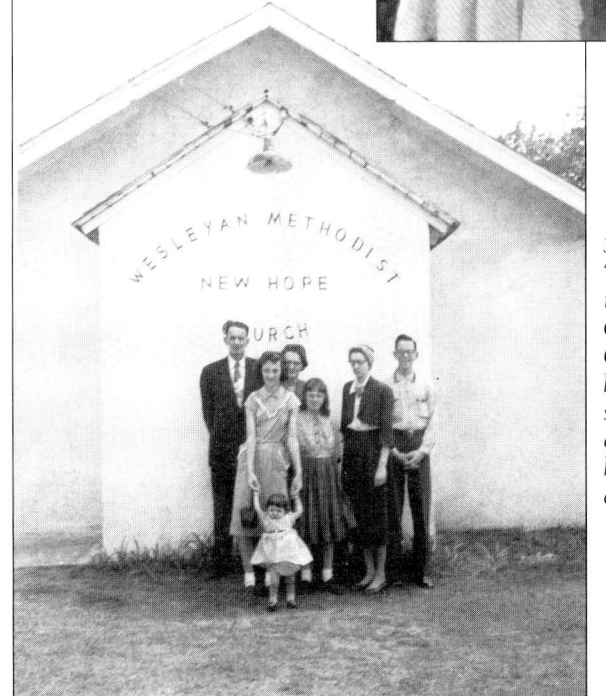

Sometime in the mid '50's, a return to our roots. The New Hope Church near Ringwood, Oklahoma. Her parents behind her on either side, the author holds onto little Jeanette, beside Lillian, Millie and Peter.

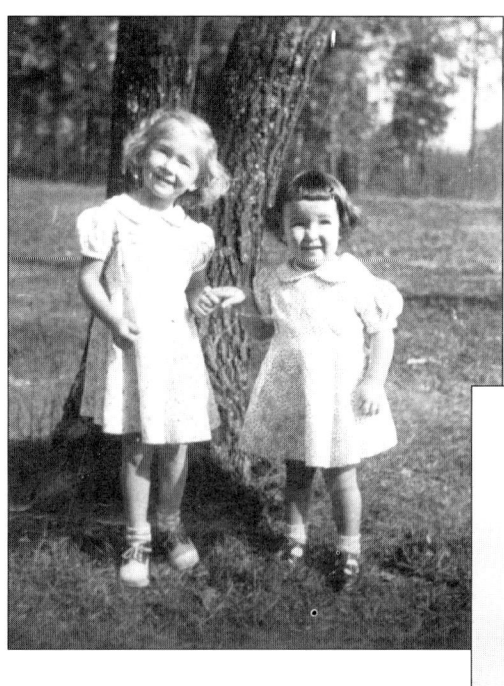

Nancy and Rosie, whose photos prompted Dad to ignore the "Don't open 'til Christmas" rule.

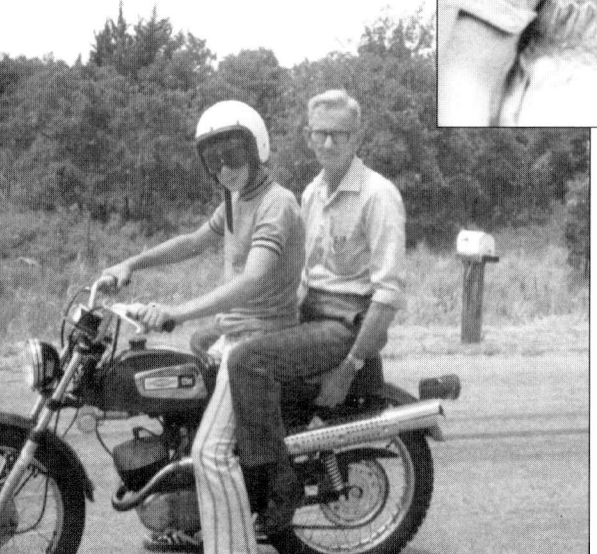

Probably the picture used to enter Lillian in the baby beauty contest.

Terry Lee with Dad, age 70.

CHAPTER THIRTEEN

Therapist or The*RAPIST*?

In the spring of 1992, eating lunch at my desk, I glanced at the blurbs capsulating articles of special interest in the local newspaper. My heart entered my throat as one line jumped out at me—"Local Christian Psychologist Cited in Sex Scandal."

"You don't suppose—you don't just suppose...."

"Nah, couldn't be," I argued with myself. "And yet...."

Ever since the Licensing Board spokesman, twelve years earlier, had asked if we had hard evidence of sexual misconduct by Dr. French, I was sure the State of Washington had received complaints against him which as yet they could not prove. Turning to the article, I wondered if his past had finally caught up with him.

A quick scan of the article confirmed to me that my old enemy was in deep trouble. The charges cited against him included engaging in sex with his patients, conducting "nude therapy" sessions, and violating clients' confidences. I found it ironic that his current legal problems resulted from his indulgence in the very sin he had accused my father of committing—sexual crimes against those entrusted to his care—and the sin my sister charged to me—divulging a confidence.

That article impacted me as nothing had since Lillian's note had blown my private world apart a dozen years before. Total and public vindication, identifying the *real* villain, stared at me from the open page. I stared back, rigid and non-functional.

The article hurtled me back in time to Dr. French's office. I relived the horror and outrage I experienced as he desecrated my father by his indictments against him. My mind reeled as I began to grasp the implications and repercussions of this one short article.

A plethora of questions raced through my mind as I teetered between laughter and tears. Had Ginny and Lillian seen this article? Would Lillian again become suicidal? Would she accuse Dr. French of betraying her as she had accused me?

Did they already know of French's indiscretions? Would they defend him? Perhaps they would not accept the report as truth. Had French preempted this publicity by giving his followers his own version of the story? Would he assume a role of martyrdom, proclaiming his innocence in the midst of persecution?

Perhaps Ginny had known about this all the while I had lived with her. Indeed, she *had* mysteriously quit going to Dr. French just prior to our invasion of their home. Did this explain her sudden termination of therapy? I had not detected in her any disillusionment concerning him. To the contrary, she had seemed gratified that her daughters and their husbands were seeing him and reaping the benefits of his "intensive therapy."

The article said he had engaged in sex with his clients. Did that include my sisters and nieces? Would they consent to such a thing? I didn't think so, but neither had I believed they would turn against their father or grandfather with such claims against him, either.

What about Lillian? Would she continue to see him if he proved to be a sexual predator, preying on those who trusted him? Wasn't that her big complaint about Dad? Would it be different now that it was her therapist under fire?

Dr. French had admitted to using nude therapy with his clients. Had this been part of my sisters' therapy? My nieces' therapy? What about the men in my family, the husbands of my nieces? Did he prescribe nude therapy for them also?

If he didn't use this form of therapy with my relatives, did they know he used it with others? Did they defend and deify him, knowing of his dubious methodologies? They attended his retreats and seminars. What went on at those events?

I was angry, angry, *angry*! How dare this diabolical opportunist point his dirty finger at my dad! No wonder he came up with such warped conclusions! He probably was incapable of entertaining a decent thought. I abhorred the fact that I had deliberately attempted to give Dr. French the benefit of the doubt over and over again, trying not to be unfair in my judgments of him. My mother was correct. I had not been nearly hard enough on him!

I was angry, but I was also concerned about what this would mean to my sisters and their families. I feared the cult-like intensity of their loyalty to Dr. French would weather any storm, even this one.

As I monitored area newspapers, a broader picture of Dr. French's activities emerged. The State Examining Board of Psychology had filed a complaint against Dr. French due to allegations that he had violated professional ethics by having sex with his patients. Of the multitude of women who had complained about his treatment, six were willing to go public. Their complaints against him were contained in the Statement of Charges.

In a letter dated April 1, 1991, written to his clientele, French confessed to having a "long-standing intimate relationship" with "one of my former clients. ...She and I came to an out-of-court compromise..." Reports put the settlement at three hundred thousand dollars.

The letter continued, "Frankly and with deep sorrow, I admit I was wrong.... It has been said I had sex with another client during Intensive in 1976. Such a claim is false."

He then told of his deep repentance and the subsequent forgiveness and restoration he had received from the Lord during his

Skeletons Without Bones

own self-administered "intensive" during January of that same year. The rest of the letter was full of his own concern lest his patients be unable to forgive him for being human like themselves and thus jeopardize their own mental, physical and spiritual well-being.

Perhaps I was unduly prejudiced, but his repentance appeared shallow and self-serving to me.

My niece Danita, entertaining doubts of her own, asked Dr. French, "Is the woman mentioned in your letter the only one?"

He assured her, "Yes, she was the only one."

She persisted, "She was the only one? I'm not going to read in the paper that you're really a 'dirty old man'?"

"Well, there was one other, just one time."

Danita accepted that. For someone less mesmerized by him, problems abounded and questions remained unanswered. What about the other women who stated under oath that he had also had sex with them—not once, but in therapy sessions every week extending over many years?

However willing some may have been to gloss over Dr. French's indiscretions, I determined I would discover the truth about him. Had I not investigated my own father? I would do no less regarding his accuser.

The Washington State Examining Board of Psychology scheduled Dr. French's hearing for June 12, 1992. My husband and I took time off work to attend the all-day event. My investigation had begun.

I couldn't help but laugh when it was announced that Dr. French would not be present at the hearing due to his age and health. Just a few days before, curious to see how a man charged with multiple counts of sexual indiscretion conducts himself in such a setting, I had attended a home Bible study led by Dr. French.

I need not have concerned myself. He obviously was among friends and had nothing to fear from them. The class was as uninspiring as it was uneventful.

The interesting part came after the class was completed. The home in which the Bible study was conducted overlooked Puget

Sound. The host had recently completed building a beautiful yacht, and invited all the guests to tour his craft.

As we filed out the door to navigate the pier, Dr. French stepped aside for me to pass and commented, "So you are Donna!"

I met his gaze and affirmed, "I am Donna."

If he remembered that morning in his office twelve years before, he gave no indication. With no evidence of the disdain with which he had formerly treated me, on this occasion he exuded nothing but grace and charm.

So it happened that I walked down the rustic stairway and along the loosely-connected slats that formed the narrow pier, escorted by a most agile and coordinated Dr. French. He was in perfect form and balance in spite of the lurching and pitching of the long floating structure under siege of a multitude of footsteps.

Upon reaching the vessel, we found that to get down into the cabin we must descend a narrow, perpendicular ship's ladder. I hesitated, wanting to see how the esteemed Doctor at age seventy-eight would navigate such a challenge. Without difficulty, without misgivings and without aid, he disappeared down the ladder with as much ease as the youngest among us.

Less than a week later, his age and health left him disinclined to attend his hearing.

I could scarcely blame him. As I looked around at the room full of people, I recognized none of his usual entourage. Even his attorney looked a mite lonely.

As the complainants took the stand, the details that emerged sounded all too familiar. Each witness acknowledged complete trust in her counselor, the more so because he claimed to be Christian. Each referred to the cult-like totalitarian atmosphere in which he operated. They admitted they had equated him with God or Jesus Christ, which reminded me of how Ginny's entire demeanor would change in his presence. Her hands would come together in front of her chest and she would walk with the floating footsteps of one who worshipped before a shrine.

One client testified that on her last day of intensive, after a session of nude therapy, Dr. French told her that he was the person who prepared the bride for the Bridegroom.

Instantly I recognized the phraseology as that used by Dr. French when he declared Dad had told Lillian the same thing, verbatim! As I listened to this woman's testimony given under oath, I realized Dr. French himself must have been the originator of the statement he had then credited to my father.

In fact, a subterranean suspicion bubbled to the surface of my mind. Perhaps Lillian's recovered memories had more substance than I had previously supposed. Could Dr. French, with a little hypnotic hocus-pocus, have scrambled the time, place, and identity of Lillian's sexual predator, even as he himself preyed upon her—body, mind and soul?

Dr. McIlroy alluded to that possibility in a letter he sent me dated November 21, 1994:

> *I have taken courses in hypnosis and have used it for preparation of patients for surgery, post-operative care, pain control...and to help patients with post-traumatic stress problems. Hypnosis is a powerful and helpful instrument but **it can be used to manipulate and injure the patient.** [Emphasis mine.]*

Himself a trained and proficient hypnotist, Dr. French cited affiliation with two professional hypnosis societies. In spite of his assurance to me that therapists do not lead or influence their clients, I possess a brochure distributed by the Hypnodyne Foundation of Clearwater, Florida, that advertises a seminar titled "Hypnotherapy Certification Weekend." It boasts that on the first day, participants will work with "fixation, relaxation, visualization and *suggestion*.... You will learn the use of *specific suggestions*." The second day, "you will learn how to formulate *effective suggestions*." [Emphasis mine.]

So much for Dr. French's claim that therapists do not intend to influence the perception and behavior of their clientele![1]

Witnesses continued to cite their complaints. They spoke of Dr. French's extreme sarcasm and verbal abuse to them when they displeased him. Some admitted they were afraid of him, stating he had threatened physical violence to at least one of them. Before taking the stand, they had requested the court to forbid TV cameras to show their faces on screen, for fear of his retribution. Throughout the hearing, their real names were never given.

The audience at the hearing consisted mainly of former clients of Dr. French, accompanied by their current therapists who were helping them recover from the therapy they had received from Dr. French. Though they were unwilling to publicly expose their own involvements—one woman said, "I am a school teacher and a mother; no way could I go public!"—these women were nevertheless offering moral and emotional support to clients brave enough to do so.

We learned much from these public testimonies, but perhaps we learned more during the breaks and at lunch time. Since I bear an obvious resemblance to my sister Ginny in looks, voice and mannerisms, many of Dr. French's former clients mistook me for her. When they learned I was not Ginny, but that I was her sister, they still accepted me as one of them. They were disappointed and concerned when they learned my sisters and my nieces remained under Dr. French's influence. They asked whether my sisters had engaged in sexual relations with Dr. French. I could only say, "I don't know—I don't think so. At least they deny any such involvement."

These sad but wiser women all nodded and said, "We would have denied it, too." Their consensus was that any female who continued long in therapy with Dr. French was likely involved with him sexually. Their conclusions were not very heartening to me.

Speaking freely around the lunch table, these former clients of Dr. French confessed that no part of their lives had escaped his influence. Some of them had adopted children, the arrangements for which were made by none other than the Doctor himself. Now, knowledge of his sexual exploits had convinced them that he doubtless had a vested interest in the parade of ever-available infants he placed into established families! One can imagine the havoc these suspicions played upon a family already ravaged by this man's unscrupulous marauding of their fidelity, their finances and their futures.

When one witness had questioned Dr. French concerning the propriety of their sexual relationship in light of the fact they were both married, his explanation was characteristically as stupid as it was self-serving. He assured her, "We are not committing adultery. In India milk became 'adulterated' when some impurity had been introduced to make it so. But when we have sex, I give to you my own 'pure love.' Something so uncontaminated could never be labeled 'adultery'."

It is not difficult to establish Dr. French's motivations, but one has to wonder at the gullibility of the women. Their mesmerization can only be understood within the concept of a cult.

At the conclusion of the six-hour hearing, two women who had been spectators during the proceedings compared notes. Both were victims of therapy abuse, though as yet they had not disclosed to each other the identity of their therapists. Finally one ventured, "I am a former patient of Dr. French. Your experience sounds almost identical to mine. Was he your therapist too?"

"No," the other woman assured her, "my therapist was a much younger man." Further comparing of notes, however, revealed the disturbing fact that the younger man had received his training from Dr. French!

One hates to guess how many of his clones are out there, eager to carry on his "tradition." And one has to wonder how many more women will allow themselves to be duped by them—or others like them—and pay lucrative fees for the privilege?

We left that hearing with a fuller knowledge of the degradation of our enemy and the scope of influence he wielded. His victims that we could identify— clients and their families—numbered well into the hundreds. We hoped we had just witnessed the beginning of the end of his little empire.

A few days following that hearing, our friend Bruce commented, "Friday morning I saw you guys in your pickup heading north. Did you take a day off work to have some fun?"

One could scarcely call attending Dr. French's hearing "fun!" I nearly brushed off the teasing question when I realized I needed to pursue this conversation to clear up an old misunderstanding.

Bruce and his wife Gwen had begun to attend the same church we belonged to. Recognizing them as friends of my sister and brother-in-law, I introduced myself to them as Ginny's sister.

Gwen had responded, "Oh, we not only know Ginny, but we know your sister Lillian as well. We even know about the incest. Lillian told us all about it."

Gwen's remark had left me stunned and outraged. I suspected that Lillian's problem with me was not that she wanted anonymity and confidentiality concerning her story, but rather that she believed she possessed "exclusive rights" to the telling of it. It seemed that she was both author and star of her personal soap-opera and in no instance would she tolerate being upstaged by a member of the supporting cast!

Ginny agreed with Lillian. "It is her story and she alone has the right to tell it to whomever she chooses, any way she chooses."

Compliance with their lop-sided rule would guarantee that no one would ever hear the story except from Lillian's point of view. I could never grant Lillian that privilege. Neither Dr. French nor my sisters grasped the fact that from the time they took me into their inner sanctum and devastated my world, I also had a story, consisting of what happened to *me*, and I possessed as much right to tell my story as she had to tell hers.

Bruce's inquiry concerning our activities the morning of Dr. French's public hearing provided the ideal opportunity to clarify some things.

"Actually, we were on our way to Dr. French's hearing," I revealed, watching for their reaction.

Bruce's wife was the one who took the bait. "You went *where*?"

"We took the day off work last Friday to attend Dr. French's hearing. You knew about the hearing?"

Dumbfounded, Gwen said, "I know all about the hearing. But why would you take time off work to attend?"

"You knew Dr. French was Lillian's counselor, didn't you?"

Her shock was total and profound. If Lillian had mentioned her doctor's name, Gwen had never caught it. "I always thought there was something fishy about that story. There was so much 'hush-hush' about it, yet she was always telling it. Whenever new people came to church, by the second or third Sunday Lillian had the newcomer backed up against a wall, giving a full account of being sexually abused by her father."

As Gwen continued, it was my turn to be astounded. "I work in the state office that for years has received the complaints against Dr. French. It is our office that investigated him and brought charges against him before the State Licensing Board. But I never suspected Lillian's 'wonderful therapist' was the sexual predator we have been tracking all these years. I certainly would have no confidence in any conclusion drawn from *his* counsel."

I learned from Gwen that Washington State's Public Disclosure Act gave interested citizens access to French's bulging file, so I took another afternoon off work to examine the contents in her office, which was the current equivalent to the office we had called years ago to check Dr. French's credentials.

If I had thought the testimonies at the hearing sounded disgustingly repetitive, the written complaints were even more so, *ad nauseam, ad infinitum.*

Whatever reasons prompted a woman to seek help from Dr. French, "all paths led to Rome." From both the written complaints and verbal testimonies, it appeared he diagnosed each client's problems to be a consequence of never experiencing "real love" from her parents. Furthermore, he claimed that each one was "uncomfortable with her own body and full of sexual hang-ups due to early sexual abuse"—usually incest by her father. Dr. French insisted that he alone could rid her of her hang-ups by means of "nude therapy" and his own "unconditional love."

The persistence of the therapist sooner or later overcame the reluctance of the patient, and off came the clothes. The resultant vulnerability of the client, coupled with the relentless pursuit of the therapist, culminated in the obvious—which to the unenlightened looks remarkably like the "bad" love she supposedly received from her father! His treatment makes as much sense as a medical doctor treating a patient who overdosed on drugs by injecting mega doses of the same drug.

The women under oath at the hearing confessed that once they yielded to intercourse, it became standard procedure for each weekly session. Since Dr. French's office was located in his home, the prosecuting attorney asked the women on the witness stand, "Where was Dr. French's wife during these trysts that took place in his office?" They replied, "She was in the house, sometimes in the kitchen baking cookies."

If a married couple went to therapy together, the presence of the woman's spouse on the premises offered no more a deterrent to Dr. French's exploits than did the close proximity of his own wife. The husband was simply dismissed one-half hour earlier than the wife. One wonders what would have happened if one of those men had discovered that for that extra half hour, he was paying his idol to have sex with his wife!

But they didn't catch on. Even among the women, each thought she was the only one. Curiously, they seemed to conclude Dr. French's behavior was immoral only when they discovered he had been intimate with other women besides themselves!

When the number of women claiming to have had sex with Dr. French every week for years on end, together with the ones who spent weekends with him in his home, are added to the woman who testified that even after she quit going to French for therapy, he would "drop over" to her house on Sunday afternoons for a little freebie!—it is little wonder the man failed to find the strength to attend his own hearing!

Besides describing their sexual relations with Dr. French, many of his female clients—both on the stand and in the letters on file—mentioned they had received large amounts of money from him. Sometimes it was a loan of several thousand dollars; sometimes a gift of ten or twenty thousand dollars "because he knew I was having a hard time financially at the time of my divorce," or "because I had been unable to work and he wanted to help." Other women mentioned substantial amounts labeled "scholarships," or "air fares." He paid for home improvements and financed mortgages. Whatever it was called, it amounted to pretty good insurance that the recipient was not likely to "rat" on him, no matter how uneasy she may have felt about the strange twist her therapy sessions had taken.

But who among us had been allowed to fault such a generous old man who so selflessly loved and served his patients? To question him was tantamount to treason, and indicated a suspicious, dirty mind.

My investigation confirmed that Dr. French was a man devoid of morals, integrity or restraint, while he presented himself as a model of all the above. He maintained total control of his clients and manipulated them mercilessly to his own advantage. He bought and courted them; he shamed, threatened, and intimidated them; he seduced and totally demoralized them. His methods were legion; his goal was singular—complete unquestioning subservience.

To substantiate the above conclusions, I submit a few quotes taken randomly from documents on file at the Washington State Department of Health.

- *French's therapy consists of tearing down a person's self, then saying "Now I am going to build you back again."*

- *I know I am not an isolated case in Dr. French's exploitive practice.*

- *Dr. French possessed a tremendous ego.*

- *I became a passive sexual object reliving all my previous sexual relationships for his benefit as voyeur.*

- *He made vague hints about financing my graduate studies and bringing my horse from——(overseas).*

- He said, "I don't want to rape you, I want you to give yourself body and soul."

- He said I was a demon-possessed complaining bitch who was so warped and crooked that I wouldn't fit into a coffin.

- She [Referring to Dr. French's sister] *is incensed and deeply shamed by what she calls "this sickening and wicked affair" and "the wider suffering that his filthy guilt inflicts upon those who love and trust him," referring of course to her brother and the subject of your investigations, Dr. John G. French.*

- I had a lot of confidence in myself and my integrity. He reduced me to feeling that I was good for nothing but the garbage heap by deliberate undermining and demeaning treatment. I did not deserve the destructive, vitriolic and vengeful attitudes and actions he portrayed.

- He told me he brought me out here and that I should stand on my head for him if that is what he wanted.

- He is very smart, very skillful, has exceptional verbal skills, is without any moral character and he is an expert hypnotist. He will be a hard fish to net. [This was from a male client.]

- [A former apprentice under Dr. French] *believes Dr. French may have a serious psychological illness and that his total lack of insight into both his problem and his damaging impact on his clients makes him unsafe to practice.*

- Within a few months after therapy began, sex became a regular part of therapy. He had intercourse with me during most of the hundreds of sessions I attended over the years.

- *Reverend ———— said that French voluntarily turned over his [ministerial] credentials when faced with complaints by parishioners of sexual exploitation. [This took place in the late 1940's on the East Coast.]*

Letters of complaint concerning Dr. French began to arrive at the investigative office in the State of Washington almost before the ink was dry on his license to practice in that state.

One cannot read the material in question without being overcome by the wretchedness of the man. The time has come for Dr. French to be exposed as the predator he is, and for the public to be alerted to the methods used by unscrupulous and harmful therapists and counselors to victimize unwary women who come to them seeking help.

CHAPTER FOURTEEN

"Unto the Third . . . Generation"

By Rosalyn J. Titus

AUTHOR'S NOTE: *When therapy becomes a vehicle for conjuring up here-to-for unremembered abuse, the entire family is thrown into an emotional tailspin that spans all living generations, and beyond. It mars relationships for decades, often for a lifetime. My niece Rosalyn was particularly affected by the contradictory characterizations of her Grandfather McGraw, creating for her a* Jekyll and Hyde *perception of him. Rose describes her confusion in the following chapter entitled "UNTO THE THIRD...GENERATION."*

Detonating an emotional bomb in a human pool four generations deep inevitably creates waves that move inexorably outward, leaving no one in the pool untouched. Not every member of our family felt the impact of Lillian's pronouncements with equal intensity—a natural consequence of age, gender, geography and emotional makeup.

I represent the third generation from John E. McGraw. Of my mother's four daughters, I experienced the greatest personal tur-

Skeletons Without Bones

moil stemming from Aunt Lillian's accusations as they reverberated throughout the family.

My place on the family tree is easy to identify. I am the second grandchild of John McGraw, the little "raven-haired Rosie" referred to in Chapter Two. "Golden-haired Nancy" made her debut twenty months before me. With my arrival, the tradition of sisterly pairing and bedroom sharing passed to the next generation.

The younger McGraw children were close in age to Nancy and me, and we always regarded them more as cousins than aunts and uncles, with the exception of Terry Lee. We reveled in the fact that we had an "Uncle Terry" nearly ten years our junior!

During most of my childhood, my father pastored churches in rural Wisconsin. Visits to Grandma and Grandpa McGraw were all too infrequent, since they lived in Upstate New York, Indiana and later, Oklahoma. My memories of the McGraw household are limited to various holidays when their house was bursting with an endless parade of babies, children, teens, aunts, uncles, in-laws and, if they could survive the mayhem, future in-laws.

To define my mother's family as a unique blending of unusual personalities would be an understatement. Choosing favorites is impossible. Circumstances have a way, however, of fostering emotional ties of lifelong loyalty and affection. If I were less sensitive to the feelings of the others who undoubtedly covet this distinction, I would identify Aunt Ginny as my favorite aunt.

Ginny came to live with us when I was three years old. We had moved to Madison the year before, when my father and his brother Lloyd felt called to establish a church in the state capital.

Several months prior to Aunt Ginny's arrival, my dad attended a Billy Graham movie. Standing in the foyer before the showing, Dad struck up a conversation with a tall, handsome young man in an Air Force uniform. From that chance meeting, Lyle Bedford began attending church at the YMCA where Dad and Uncle Lloyd were holding services.

No one could have predicted that by reaching out to a lonely young airman, Dad had discovered not just another "lost soul," but a lifelong soul mate. Both men were unorthodox, creative thinkers who enjoyed each other's company until my father's death in 1987.

Dad wasn't the only one with a personal liking for this young man. My mother took an interest in him "right off the bat" and put her spiritual arms around him. Four decades later, their mutual respect and affection is as strong as ever.

It is little wonder Lyle began courting Aunt Ginny soon after she arrived at our home. She was nineteen, tall and beautiful with fair skin and long dark hair. I especially remember a navy blue taffeta circle skirt she used to wear which emphasized her small waist and excellent figure.

Thanks to Dad's interest in photography, we have pictorial documentation of their romance. Throughout our childhood, Nancy and I delighted in viewing the slides of Ginny and Lyle sitting on our couch reading poetry together. While we were not above giggling at this phenomenon, we recognized something deliciously romantic about it as well.

Before long a wedding was being planned—my introduction to the mysteries of love and marriage. My mother made Aunt Ginny's long white satin gown, Uncle Lloyd performed the ceremony and my father was soloist. I have only a four-year-old's memory of Aunt Ginny's wedding. My cousin Darlene and I were low to the ground, closer to the hem of her garment than anything else. At the reception, Darlene caressed the bottom of Aunt Ginny's wedding gown, discovering an appealing substitute for the satin blanket she usually held as she sucked her thumb. Seeing the underside of the gown, I made my own shocking discovery. Aunt Ginny's fairy-tale dress was soiled where it had swept across the floor!

I have a few other memories of this early period of my life. One unforgettable day Aunt Ginny and Uncle Lyle took "just me" to a parade in which Lyle participated. Standing along the street with Aunt Ginny watching the men in uniform march past, I was disappointed that I was unable to recognize Lyle from among the dozens of military look-alikes.

Skeletons Without Bones

Another cherished memory consists of Nancy and me lying on top of the bed in Ginny and Lyle's first apartment while our new uncle told us fascinating stories, illustrating them with pictures of mythical animals which were composites of lions, horses, birds, and other creatures.

Before long Ginny and Lyle moved away from Madison to settle in Washington State, Lyle's home. Even a distance of two thousand miles could not diminish the bond between our families. Mom was always Aunt Ginny's special big sister, while Dad and Lyle would forever be kindred spirits.

We made our first trip to Seattle to visit the Bedfords in 1962, the year that city hosted the World's Fair. As a twelve-year-old catching my first glimpse of the Space Needle, I could not have imagined that the sight of this unique landmark would one day become commonplace. It is part of the magnificent view from Queen Anne High School where four years later I would begin my junior year.

During our second trip to Washington State in 1964, we spent several days camping on Spirit Lake. We have a photograph Dad took of Aunt Ginny with the awe-inspiring beauty of Mount St. Helens' snow-covered peak towering in the background. What appeared gloriously immovable that day would, two decades later, become an ash-covered wasteland, visible proof that mountains can indeed be removed and "cast into the sea." But in 1964, that was an inconceivable aspect of an unknown future.

I wish I had a mountain
A hundred miles away,
Where all the snow in my backyard
Would go and stay and stay.

That bit of doggerel, penned by my father, became reality for our family in 1966. Our two brief visits to Washington State had convinced Dad that his next move should be west.

"Unto the Third . . . Generation"

Ginny and Lyle had spent the summer of '66 traveling throughout the Midwest visiting relatives. August found them in Wisconsin, helping us with the Big Move. Our caravan westward included Lyle's van, a camper-trailer, and our family sedan pulling another trailer piled high with all of our earthly possessions.

Somehow, amid the boxes, books, bedding and other belongings, we managed to find space for four adults, two teenagers and six children. The more responsible members of our party quickly learned that making a head count after each stop was imperative.

With the current trend of remembering events that never happened, it *is* possible that some child in our company will recall being abandoned at a remote roadside rest stop in a western state, and consequently was raised by wolves. If this event someday surfaces in someone's therapy, we sincerely apologize to the wolves.

To the best of my knowledge—and with the aid, no doubt, of at least a dozen (one each) guardian angels—we all arrived safely in Seattle shortly before the new school year began.

Our family stayed with Ginny and Lyle until Dad found a job and permanent housing. Needless to say, we spent a great deal of time together that first year.

With the commencement of our second year in Seattle, Lyle took a teaching position in another city. Over the next two decades we faithfully contributed to the increasing traffic congestion on the stretch of freeway between Seattle and Ginny's house.

Most holidays found us celebrating together, and Sunday afternoon drives to Ginny's house were not uncommon. During these visits the Bedford cousins and my two younger sisters, Joanne and Patsy, entertained themselves with Barbies or board games or more boisterous amusements. By contrast, Nancy and I, advancing beyond adolescence into our late teens and early twenties, became a rapt audience for the stimulating discussions engendered by Mom, Ginny, Dad and Lyle.

As often as not, their conversations evolved from the most recent book, article or sermon one of them had read or heard. Topics were as diverse as theology, politics, parenting, nutrition, person-

Skeletons Without Bones

ality types and marriage. Opinions were freely and lavishly put forth and literally ranged from the sublime to the ridiculous.

Nancy and I reaped personal benefits from this periodic exposure to and exploration of new ideas and concepts. We became less satisfied with superficial thinking and learned to express ourselves with more maturity and insight than might otherwise have been the case. We both felt we were acquiring at least a modicum of intellectual sophistication.

When in the course of time Aunt Ginny's conversational contributions began to include insights from her new guru and spiritual guide, we saw nothing insidious or unusual about this. Coming from Ginny, the advent of an enlightened version of Christianity-cum psychology was as normal and unremarkable as the eventual appearance of tuna fish sandwiches and jello salad on her vast kitchen table. Food and philosophy were frequently served up together. One way or another, we were being fed.

I have been intrigued by psychology and why people are the way they are for as long as I can remember. Because I was interested in helping people and understanding their problems, I became a sponge around Ginny and Lillian. During my twenties and thirties no one in my sphere of influence spoke with such great conviction about the cause, effect and answers to deep psychological problems.

I never doubted that these two intelligent and well-read women were also truth seekers. For years they both wholeheartedly received and embraced counsel from Dr. French. For more than twenty years, from the early 1970's until 1992, I had no hint from either Ginny, Lillian, or their children—several of whom by now were under his professional care—that there was any reason to question Dr. French or the efficacy of his therapy.

They spoke of Dr. French in tones of awe and reverence. His word constituted gospel and he was placed on a level of integrity equal to my godly grandfathers who were honest, sincere Bible-believing Christian ministers. As a matter of fact, Dr. French was usually depicted as being a cut above most pastors and teachers. His wisdom and enlightenment had surpassed the supposed "immature, naive and even clown-like" doctrines of the churches in which most of us had been reared and to which most of the family still adhered.

I had no reason to doubt this doctor or his theology, especially since his "truth" had helped Ginny and "cured" Lillian, when all other truths and teachers had apparently failed. So for years I listened and believed, on the basis of Ginny and Lillian's testimony of their healing and their adulation of their healer, that the polish they put on the apple represented whole and uncorrupted fruit.

With the information I gleaned from listening to my aunts, the never-ending analyses and unravelling of their problems seemed to follow a logical path. Wouldn't common sense suggest that the more lengthy the therapy, the more severe must be the exposed trauma? This sounded reasonable and I accepted it at face value. That Lillian's healing evolved into a decades-long process lent credence to the notion that hers was one of the more exclusive and noteworthy emotional disorders in human experience.

In light of current psychological theories, it had the ring of credibility. The concept of repressed memories appeared valid because it could account for many inexplicable neuroses, as well as the need for years of therapy—years to dig up and uncover the "memories"; additional years to determine the pervasive and venomous effect of the repressed evil; and even more years to administer the cleansing antidote.

Throughout all this time, I listened to Lillian's incessant and detailed monologues about her lifelong self-loathing. I listened first of all because failure to sympathize with her meant that you were inflicting her with the very poison that her therapist was so diligently trying to eradicate; and second, because I believed I was vicariously gaining valuable insight into the human psyche and behavior.

Lillian always spoke with such great conviction, such undisputed intelligence and with so much information, there seemed to be no solid basis for questioning her insights. But the factor that gave her illness and its cure so much credibility was the unquestionable integrity of her therapist.

One Wednesday in April of 1992, I chanced to pick up a copy of the Seattle *Times* after work. Giving it a cursory going-over as I walked home, a column headline on the front page caught my attention—*Local Psychologist Implicated in Sex Scandal*.

As I read the article, thinking, "It couldn't be Dr. French," I was shocked to find that it was, indeed, the esteemed doctor.

"Anybody can be accused..." I countered, my indoctrination coming to his defense. But after reading a full-length column on the front page, and continuing with several more columns on page two, it was clear that this was no vague, isolated accusation in its embryonic stages.

Several women had made accusations claiming that Dr. French had sex with them during therapy. An out-of-court settlement of $300,000 already had been paid to one of these former patients. In addition, Dr. French had made a statement admitting he was "wrong and in violation of his professional ethics."

I don't claim to have a brilliant legal mind, but when multiple accusations are made and a sizeable monetary settlement is agreed upon and paid, that strikes me as either an admission of guilt or an attempt to stifle further investigation. However disbelieving I might feel, I could not simply shrug this off as unfounded allegations. Suddenly, because of the random purchase of a local newspaper, I found myself compelled to reconsider the light in which I had been viewing the supposed skeletons in the family closets.

So great was my agitation and astonishment after finishing the article, I set aside my usual frugality and called my mother in Florida without waiting for evening or weekend rates. Mom had always been a confidante to Ginny and had maintained the lines of communication with Lillian. Therefore I felt she should be informed about what I was reading in the *Times*.

I assumed that since the story was just now breaking in the state's largest newspaper, it could not long remain a secret from Dr. French's clientele. How could Aunt Ginny and Aunt Lillian fail to hear something so openly proclaimed and remain unaffected by it? Wasn't it likely that when Ginny and Lillian learned of this fall-from-grace of their long-time mentor and spiritual guide, they would be shocked and devastated? In my naiveté I believed my mother should be prepared to counsel and comfort them in the near future.

As days and then weeks passed, however, nothing was heard from either Ginny or Lillian in response to this scandal. Surely they couldn't be in the dark about these reports. That was so improbable that a new possibility began to emerge: maybe the sex scandal involving their doctor was old news to them. This unexpected reticence may have been their *modus operandi* for longer than the rest of the family could have imagined.

If that were the case, it seemed unconscionable that they could choose to ignore the sins of their therapist, when for years they had been supporting his unproven theories about their own father's supposed immorality. There had been no inhibitions on Lillian's part about proclaiming Grandpa's "evil deeds" to anyone who would sympathetically listen. Why then this deafening silence when the renowned therapist's immorality was exposed?

Then again, does it really matter?

Grandpa is dead. Lillian claims to be well. Dr. French has admitted to falling off his pedestal. And the family seems able to congenially communicate and congregate.

What more could you wish? What could be gained by stirring up old misunderstandings, once again risking dissention? What justification could be made for sucking up the iridescent covering of oil and re-troubling the family waters?

What, indeed, could you possibly gain?

The truth—that's all! Truth is a rock, providing a solid foundation. Falsehood and error are sand, shifting and unstable.

For years the cousins in my generation have been confronted with two opposing and totally contradictory claims to Truth. And for twenty years I have been sitting on the fence between the two.

But now the ground is beginning to shake and I must decide which way to jump. Which side is rock? Which is sand? Is there any way to discover which is which, or must I take a blind leap in the dark?

CHAPTER FIFTEEN

The Elephant in the Living Room

During the months we monitored the continuing saga of Dr. French's escapades, an equally fascinating and definitely more pleasurable drama was unfolding within the ranks of our family. An impromptu family reunion was miraculously taking shape.

In recent alternate years we had held reunions attended by about half of the McGraw children and a fourth of the grandchildren. The last gathering had taken place in Texas the previous year, with the next one scheduled for 1993.

However, Mother was experiencing increasing forgetfulness, which she feared would soon render her incapable of recognizing her children and grandchildren. So the spring of 1992 found different ones of us, starting with Anna, independently making plans to visit Mother in Edinburg, Texas, where she lived with my sister Millie.

As word spread that various brothers and sisters were making arrangements to visit Mom, the proverbial snowball began to gather momentum. Grandchildren started making plans. Soon we all began looking for ways to stretch budgets to include a trip to see Grandma McGraw. To accommodate the growing numbers, the location was changed. The church property in Kansas where Louise's husband pastored was spacious enough, and the local congregation gracious enough, to accommodate the seventy-some potential attendees.

The airlines gave the final impetus to our plans by cutting fares in half. Phone lines hummed as families who had expected to buy tickets at full price now arranged to buy twice as many at half price, thus enabling all of Mother's thirteen children (counting Lottie, who came to us full-grown), eight of their spouses, and large numbers of grandchildren and great-grandchildren, to celebrate together her eighty-fourth birthday.

We watched awe-struck as the marvelous occasion took shape. The inclusion of aunts, uncles, cousins and close friends heightened our delight. We were convinced that the Lord had arranged the whole affair for us all, but especially for Mother. We could not name another time we had all been together; we knew we were uncommonly blessed.

Millie's daughter Esther Ruth, the granddaughter with whom our parents had lived in Puerto Rico, was scheduled to leave the following winter for her first term as a missionary teacher in Malaysia. She had dreamed of having her seldom-seen extended family participate in her commissioning service. We now scheduled that service to take place the Sunday evening of our reunion. Could we doubt the Lord's handiwork in fulfilling her dream beyond what she could ask or think?

Our time together recaptured some of the hilarity of our large, fun-filled family. With private rooms at a premium, young families with babies were given the preferred accommodations. Many of the rest of us stayed together in dormitory-like arrangements. The basement of the church served as men's dorm while the women occupied the upstairs of the parsonage. This may not have been considered ideal at first glance, but it was nevertheless reminiscent of the unavoidable sharing of facilities we had known as kids at home. It also provided the women opportunity for intimate girl-talk. I am ignorant of what men do in their quarters in such circumstances.

As families came and went during the course of our week in Kansas, much-prized private rooms sometimes became available, eliciting some good-natured vying and jockeying for dibs on newly-vacated space.

On one occasion, Millie preempted any bargaining by staking claim to the most recent vacancy. She claimed her husband Bill showed signs of elevated blood pressure, and she felt he would rest better in a more secluded arrangement.

Out-maneuvered by Millie, the rest of us girls made our way to our makeshift dorm. We were in our night clothes, fixing hair, reading and talking, when a rejected Millie came dragging back into the common room to reclaim her former bunk. Having secured rights to the coveted accommodations, she had sallied forth to report her victory to her awaiting husband, only to find him sound asleep in the men's quarters! Amidst our ribbing, she returned to her roost, reluctantly relinquishing rights to room and romance to rivaling relatives.

In a few minutes my husband's voice wafted up the stairway, calling my name. In that moment, with the eyes of my sisters, sisters-in-law and nieces on me, I swept past them, making the most of my exit. At the door, I turned and giggled my confession.

"I can't help it! I feel exactly as if I were Esther, chosen from among the harem to be the Queen."

Amidst their howls of protest I went to meet my astonished husband who had no clue as to what had precipitated such bedlam emanating from the women's quarters!

It was a healing time for our family. No one spoke openly of the accusations toward our father that had divided us over the past decade. We were intent on reaffirming our love and commitment to one another. Almost we could forget the deep schism that had threatened to rend us apart.

Sunday afternoon as we finished our mid-day meal, my brother John stood to his feet. Soon he and his family would have to leave, but first he wanted to say a few words. Addressing his remarks to

Mom, he delivered the most touching tribute to a mother and dad I have ever heard. In his down-home manner, John thanked her for taking him as a baby and raising him as her own. He spoke of the love and security he had experienced in spite of the challenge that school presented to him. He spoke of reconnecting with his birth family in his adult years, producing an even deeper appreciation for the home in which he had been reared.

After John's well-spoken remarks, others of the children just naturally followed. Mother's step-daughters, her adopted children, her sons- and daughters-in-law, and her birth children joined together in expressing their love and appreciation for her and Dad.

No cassettes recorded those eulogies as far as I know; they came too spontaneously to have been anticipated. But John's reverie spawned a never-to-be-forgotten tribute to a most deserving woman and her late husband.

Almost we could forget the breach that separated us. Almost it was as if it had never happened.

Almost—but not quite. Because some, influenced by Dr. French's slander of John and Opal McGraw, decided that the whole event had been orchestrated, staged by the "Loyalists" for the benefit of the "French Quarter." They could not imagine that kind of regard just naturally overflowing from the hearts of the offspring of a couple as degenerate as Dr. French had concocted.

Almost forgotten was the rift—but not quite. For Lillian was offended because we could all praise and honor Mother and Daddy, but she didn't feel free to openly eulogize her Dr. French!

Almost forgotten were the damaging untruths—but not quite. For while we were viewing old family slides, a discussion ensued as to the identity of the person holding aloft baby Terry Lee for a close-up shot.

The query, "Is that Mother?" elicited a pointed response from my next-younger sister, "No! She never took care of Terry Lee!"

Spontaneously, I quietly objected, "That's not true!" Seated on the sofa next to me, my niece Rose asked, "What did you say?"

I repeated my muted declaration, "That's not true. That's ridiculous! Of course Mom took care of Terry."

The Elephant in the Living Room

Lillian and Dr. French had fashioned a virtual Cinderella out of Lillian. She supposedly was the ill-treated little waif who was forced or shamed into doing all the house-cleaning and all the child-care of the younger children. Reminiscent of the better-known fairy tale, Cinder-lillian stayed home and worked while we ugly older sisters went out and had all the fun.

Lillian claimed she sometimes worked almost all night long, cleaning the house while the rest of us lazy slobs slept. And what about Mother? She did nothing but sit around all day.

Come to think of it, Lillian is the only one of us with feet small enough to wear a dainty glass slipper!

Rose had heard the above stories, and other similar ones, all her adult life. Now at age forty, sitting on the sofa at a family reunion, for the first time she heard someone actually refute one of Lillian's tirades. Since Rose had so recently found out the truth about Dr. French, she listened with both ears!

Ostensibly, we had left Dr. French thousands of miles back in Washington State; in reality, his unwelcome influence invaded our almost perfect family gathering.

Once again, what we heard from the French Quarter was a distortion of real events. In truth, Lillian often took care of the younger children, neither by mandate nor coercion, but rather by her own preference. She loved the babies and enjoyed taking care of them. After school, she habitually darted upstairs to our room where the youngest member of our brood would be waking from a nap. Lillian would dress the child and bring him or her downstairs where the action was.

So consistently did Lillian adhere to this pattern that one time I incurred her wrath because I had the audacity to dress the baby before she arrived home! She informed me that was her job and just because I arrived home first did not give me license to encroach upon her prerogatives!

One summer the community held a doll and pet show at our local elementary school. Lillian dressed dainty little Jeanette and her equally dainty little doll in their Sunday best and took them to the school so Jeanette could enter her doll in the contest.

Lillian brought the doll home adorned with a blue ribbon. But her proudest moment had occurred when one of the judges lifted Jeanette to the table, and sitting her among the "other dolls," declared her to be the prettiest of all!

Force Lillian to take care of the children? There would have been neither opportunity nor necessity to do so. For as long as I can remember, Lillian was an eager "little mother" by her own inclination and volition.

Is it any wonder I was dumbfounded when years later I was confronted with the accounts of how Lillian was forced to take care of the babies because Mother neglected to do so?

Just as the events leading to our reunion had run concurrently with the Dr. French saga, so the culmination of both events occurred simultaneously. The final day of our reunion I received a phone call from our friend Gwen back in Washington State confirming that the Psychology Review Board had found Dr. French guilty of unethical conduct. They barred him from renewing his license for twenty years and fined him the maximum amount allowed by existing laws, the largest fine ever leveled by that body against a psychologist in the State of Washington.

On our flight home, my niece Rose observed, "Yes, it was a good reunion. But we never addressed the real issue. It is the proverbial elephant in the middle of the living room, but we all ignore it, pretending it is not there."

Chapter Sixteen

The Family Fights Back

Following the 1992 reunion, we all returned to our homes, taking with us the lingering knowledge that we had participated in a miracle. Yet Lillian's remark accusing Mother of never taking care of Terry Lee still rankled in my ears.

The time approached when we would have to evict the elephant from our living room. To that end, I tried to encapsulate on paper the sentiment expressed around the dinner table that Sunday afternoon at our reunion. We, the children of John and Opal McGraw, had too long tolerated the scurrilous attacks upon our parents from within our ranks. The document I drafted declared that each of the undersigned children witnessed and testified to our parents' exemplary lives. It attested that Dr. French had proven himself an unworthy and unreliable source of counsel and information; we wanted to hear no more of him.

After I completed the draft of this *Document of Defense*, I put it away, ready to retrieve it at the appropriate time.

That fall of 1992 Lillian turned fifty. Plans were afoot to give her a big surprise party in her own home. To allow opportunity for the festive preparations, I was assigned responsibility for luring her from the premises for the entire day.

Lillian and I spent a fun day shopping, returning that evening to a darkened house that gave no clue as to what awaited her. One step inside her kitchen, however, revealed a house full of well-wishers and all the trappings of an "over-the-hill" celebration.

Lillian responded with surprise and delight. I, however, stood rooted to the spot in horrified shock. In the living room against the far wall sat none other than my old adversary, looking hale and hearty—apparently recovered from whatever ailment prevented his appearance at his hearing five months before—and accepting as his just due all the hugs and kisses lavished upon him by my adoring relatives!

Betrayed and outraged, I tried to determine what my proper response should be. I was repulsed at being forced to socialize with the man who had labeled my father a sexual pervert; who had ripped our family apart while he used the confidentiality of his office to play the gigolo.

In disgust I watched as Dr. French received the honor and affection that had been denied my father in his final years. And I remembered Mom describing Daddy's last visit to Washington State when, in the gathering fog of Alzheimer's disease, he wept in bed at night as he suffered the rejection of his youngest daughter who refused to see him. Whether he ever comprehended the indictment she had leveled against him, I do not know.

My determination increased to make it clear that Dr. French's status was *persona non grata* to me and much of the rest of the family.

Four months following her birthday party, Lillian was visiting my niece Rose, and seized the opportunity to climb back up on her soap box. "Mother never held me or told me she loved me. I was spanked every day."

People who merely play the role of a survivor of incest, as is true of all entertainers, must keep coming up with new material in order to maintain the interest of their audiences. Lillian failed to realize she had already lost this audience.

For a year Rose had been trying to sort out and discard all the false information she had received from her Aunt Lillian. To be regaled with new allegations, this time against her grandmother, was more than Rose could tolerate.

Did this new attack on Mother signal that the time had come to unveil my statement of defense? I read the rough draft to Rose, and later to Anna, both of whom promptly sanctioned it as a reasonable course of action.

We finalized the statement, made copies, and sent it on its way for signatures. As the document made the rounds among family members, I contacted three long-standing friends, and asked them to write for Lillian a description of how they remembered her as a young girl and as a teenager.

Late that summer, when Anna was in Washington for a visit, we delivered our statement of defense, along with copies of the requested letters from friends, to Lillian and three nieces visiting her at the time.

In the presence of the girls, Anna explained our mission to Lillian, offering them each a copy of the material we had collected. We vouched for Daddy's innocence, stating, "We are speaking on behalf of Mother and the other brothers and sisters who have signed this document."

Incensed, Lillian and the girls refused the envelopes, declaring, "We won't read it. Why are you dragging this all up again. After all, Grandpa is long gone and this is a dead issue."

"No," we countered. "It is not a dead issue. It has never been resolved and Lillian continues to talk about it at every opportunity. Now she is adding new charges against grandmother and we are no longer putting up with such tirades against our parents.

A heated discussion followed, during which Lillian assumed her "poor Cinderella" role and the girls rallied to her defense. "Everybody, including good parents, have faults and failures," they said. "Why can't you admit that even though your dad was a good man, he was not perfect; he made a mistake?

Lillian chimed in, "The sexual thing lasted only about a year, when I was very small, about eighteen months old. It never happened after that."[1]

Whoa! Red flags went up in my head. There were all kinds of things wrong with that statement. I didn't have time to analyze it all then, but I grasped at one inconsistency.

"Only one year? Never again? What about your story that you hated to sit on Dad's lap in the car on the way to Baldwinsville? You said when you did, Dad had an erection and it felt like you were sitting on a stick. That was not when you were little! That was ten or twelve years later!"

Lillian admitted, "Yes, that was much later."

Pressing my advantage, I continued, "We are not talking about a slight problem or failure here. We're talking about one of the most heinous crimes one person can commit against another. We are talking about something for which Dad could have spent years behind bars."

"Oh, no," she assured me. "I would never have sent him to jail!"

Was she unaware the law requires such crimes to be reported to the authorities? Dr. McIlroy had indicated he would have done so had he seen anything amiss. Did she not know that authorities must investigate each report, and that investigations often resulted in costly law suits and lengthy jail sentences? Had she ever considered what her accusations meant to anyone other than herself?

Finally Lillian had heard enough. "My family never did love and accept me," she declared. "This confrontation is just further evidence of that fact. You can continue this discussion without me if you choose, but I have a child to feed and other important things to do."

With that, she left. I expected the girls to follow her lead (as I suspect Lillian likewise expected), but they did not. Instead, Danita confessed she had never before heard the incident about Lillian sitting on Dad's lap in the car. I countered that many aspects of the story she had never heard because she had chosen to listen only to Lillian, and Lillian was selective in what she told whom.

Arriving at an inconclusive conclusion, Anna and I prepared to leave Lillian's house, the envelopes containing the rejected copies of the *Document of Defense* still in our possession.

It was an awkward departure. Anna would soon be returning home to Florida and farewells were in order. She had long been a protector of Lillian and the closest and favorite aunt to these three nieces as they grew up. She had also been a defender of their therapist, and as far as I knew, of Lillian's complete story. For Anna to openly challenge Lillian and Dr. French could not help but have an impact upon them.

Lillian joined us outside as we said our goodbyes out in the yard. She once again declared her family as typically uncaring and rejecting of her. But somehow she ended up in Anna's embrace and they stood a long time with their arms around each other. Anna reassured her that this was a not a rejection of her person. It was a repudiation of her untrue memories and charges. Since those for whom we had prepared our defense refused to receive it, its impact appeared to score somewhere between zero and zilch. Even so, Anna was confident we had done the right thing and was content to leave the results to the Lord.

My own response was less spiritual and completely pessimistic. My faith had plummeted to its lowest level. I could not even make myself produce copies of the spurned material, despite my promise to send a copy to each signer. I was tired of the fight, burned out on the topic, and disgusted with the outcome.

I could not fathom how even the Lord could produce results out of nothing. I had lost sight of the fact that "in the beginning" He had succeeded quite well in producing remarkable results out of nothing!

CHAPTER SEVENTEEN

A Declaration of Defense

The document we prepared in defense of Mother and Dad deserves a place in this account of our family's journey through the nether regions of fabricated "recovered repressed memories." It is presented here exactly as it was submitted to each adult descendant of my parents.

A DECLARATION OF DEFENSE
TO WHOM IT MAY CONCERN:

We, the undersigned children and grandchildren of John E. McGraw and Opal P. Cummings McGraw, do wish to attest to and verify the godly, consistent and unblemished character, both in conduct and teaching, of both of our above-mentioned parents.

We have no experience or knowledge, personal or otherwise, of any deviant behavior or fallacious, non-Biblical teaching by them; any mistreatment of any child, their own or children of their acquaintance; any neglect or abuse of any kind or in any degree—neither sexual, physical or otherwise; any taking of improper liberties; nor any neglect of intervention when such intervention would have been appropriate for the sake of a child.

To the contrary, we testify to the superior love, care, guidance and sense of security we experienced in our home, with both parents modeling consistent godly character of the highest degree. No child was shown either more or less love from our parents than the others. No child was undercared for or over-punished. Abuse was not present. No child was expected to carry an undue load of work or responsibilities. Mother worked hard—unhampered by speed!!—cooking, doing laundry, washing dishes, cleaning, but mostly mothering and nurturing—being there for her children and carrying the burdens and concerns of each one, all the while suffering from arthritic pain of who-knows-how-much intensity. We honestly do not know how she did it; we do not believe we could have done it; and we love and honor her for it.

Likewise Daddy was a hard-working, devoted Father who gladly clothed, housed, fed, nurtured, shepherded, and in innumerable ways provided for his large household to the best of his ability, ofttimes at the personal sacrifice of his own needs and desires. Money was never plentiful; many times it was all too scarce. Again, we stand in amazed wonder that he did so much with so little, so well. We love him and unashamedly revere his memory.

With knowledge of allegations contrary to the sentiments previously stated, and having had twelve years to think extensively; to recall memories of childhood and early years; to compare experiences; to inquire of personal friends and family acquaintances; and to investigate alleged situations and circumstances:

We, the undersigned, believe it is time to go on record to affirm that we strongly regret, resent and refute any and all such allegations and attacks on the unblemished lives and characters of our duly loved and esteemed parents, and also on other members of our family similarly accused. We do hereby desire to clear Father's good name and to attest Mother's faultless demeanor and to give them the honor and respect they thoroughly deserve. We do this not only for their sake and our own, but for the sake of the grandchildren and great-grandchildren who so desperately need to know, appreciate and emulate the remarkable models and the heritage that is rightfully theirs in Grandma and Grandpa McGraw.

We strongly regret any and all circumstances and choices that have precipitated such charges as have been made, and we do willingly and unreservedly extend our love and sympathy to any and all who for whatever reasons believe otherwise and have therefore been robbed of a precious heritage. We know of no valid foundation for such conclusions. We regret the severe pain, trauma and alienation that such a position has generated in the persons who have taken this position. We similarly and just as strongly regret the severe pain, trauma and alienation it has produced in the lives of those who openly opposed that position.

We, the undersigned, do violently and completely regret, resent and refute all the unfounded, ridiculous, insidious, slanderous conclusions leveled against our parents by one former psychologist, namely John George French. We find it particularly significant and repulsive that said psychologist has found himself embroiled in a much-publicized sex scandal of immense proportions, and has been found guilty of numerous counts of sexual misconduct and has been denied a license by the State of Washington's Department of Health Licensing Board.

This unconscionable behavior was obviously being perpetrated by John French at the very time he was leveling accusations at our Father, and indirectly at our Mother. Since things done in secret have indeed been shouted from the rooftops, e. g., media headlines and national TV exposés, we will no longer stand mutely by when John French is eulogized and adulated and/or our parents are accused, attacked and maligned. John French has completely discredited himself and destroyed any credibility he may have appeared to have.

Wishing to put behind us the above-mentioned divisive circumstances, we declare and extend our love to all family members. We do not ask for unwilling signatures, nor do we hold animosity toward any who for any reason wish not to sign this document. This is merely an expression of the felt concerns and emotions of the undersigned children and grandchildren.

We further state our willingness to discuss the issues mentioned in this document with whomever desires such, as long as all parties involved are treated with love, respect and consideration; and as long as it is recognized and understood that the undersigned enter into such discussions holding the aforementioned positions regarding the lives and conduct of our parents.

With the document we sent the following guidelines:

- Read the document carefully. If you want to sign it as is, please do so. This is for all family members who wish to be included. If after reading it carefully, you decide it is not for you, please pass it on to the next person on the list. You may add your comments or you may add complete documents of your own. We want this to be a complete file that will include everything everyone has wanted to say. We are not trying to attack persons; we are trying to stop persons from making attacks on our parents, at least in the presence of those of us who know

A Declaration of Defense

better. And we are trying to expose the truth. We are coming out of the closet!

- The material enclosed is a combination of what various family members felt might be pertinent to the situation. Copy any parts of it you desire.

- The whole thing will be presented to the French Factor, hopefully this summer. We want to do it carefully and prayerfully. It will not be without trauma, but we think that only the knowledge and acknowledgement of truth will bring true healing, something which twenty years of falsehoods has not produced.

CHAPTER EIGHTEEN

Trapped in the Trappings

When a person taps into what he or she believes to be "recovered repressed memories," that persons's life is catapulted into a downward spiral from which few ultimately and completely recover. Masquerading as a golden gateway to mental, emotional and physical health, the search for forgotten trauma is in reality a trap door which drops the seeker into a living hell. It sucks entire families into its vortex, devastating three or four generations and predestining unborn descendants to grow up in fragmented households.

When a woman client succeeds in producing a memory, the therapy crowd rewards her with the title "survivor."[1] She is ignorant of the fact she has exchanged reality for the privilege of becoming a hollow exoskeleton, doomed to stagger under her imaginary burden, echoing the therapist's ugly edict: *Incest, incest, incest....*

Since my sister had embraced a completely skewed perception of her childhood, in an effort to help her recapture her true past I asked a few close friends to write their memories of our family in general, and of Lillian in particular. Their responses, and some old family letters, authenticate the childhood Lillian so senselessly had spurned.

The first letter comes from Faye Conley. Faye's husband pastored Willett Memorial Wesleyan Church in Syracuse, New York, where we attended from 1948 through 1957. During those years, the Conley's only child, Joy, was Lillian's best friend.

Dated July 29, 1993, Mrs. Conley began her letter by saying she had recently visited with a mutual friend from our Syracuse days. Addressing Lillian, she wrote:

> *I was telling Joy about it and we got to recalling some of the Syracuse people and events. One was when we had a quartet of four very cute little girls from the church who sang together so well and the fun we had practicing and singing.*
>
> *Donna called me recently and said you both live in Washington. My youngest sister lives in Bellevue. We have visited them twice—it is beautiful country!... If we could visit you and Donna we would have a great time recalling past days and events. I remember you and Joy being such happy little girls playing, playing and playing and having lots of fun—sometimes at the parsonage and sometimes, really more often, at your home. I was so busy with many church related activities, so we were very thankful that your Mom was so kind and generous with making Joy welcome at your home. We felt fortunate to have a church family that was so gracious and kind to our little girl.*
>
> *I recall you were two happy, giggly little girls. Some of your favorite things were playing house and playing doctor. Sometimes Marjorie and Elizabeth joined you two.... I remember going on picnics, just the four of us, and how we enjoyed seeing and being with you two happy little girls. We have many happy memories of our years at Syracuse.... We send our love and prayers. [Signed] Faye Conley.*

Joy also enclosed a letter dated July 25, 1993, addressed to Lillian.

> How happy I am to write to you after all these years. Donna called to chat and I decided to sit down and write you a few lines. Since graduating from Houghton in 1965, I have taught first grade and third grade in Corning and Horseheads, New York. I married at 45—NEVER thought it would happen—to a wonderful man, Ken Squires. He is the eldest of seven kids....
>
> It is so nice to be around a big family. Reminds me of yours when I was a kid from first thru fifth grade. I direct our choir at the Elmira Wesleyan Church where Dad came after Syracuse. Boy, was it hard to adjust to Elmira after having so many friends in Syracuse. I didn't have anyone like you to spend my hours with playing, making fudge, playing chess and SINGING! Oh, yes, did I love our quartet! Are you still singing?
>
> It is with great happiness I recall our years of friendship. Our intimate talks about boys—(remember the Zoble boys, Gene and Howard?)
>
> You were my best friend, you know. Please write and tell me how you are! I would LOVE to hear from you! We may be separated by thousands of miles but only thoughts away. Please write!
>
> [Signed] Joy Conley Squires.

Lillian's original note written to me accusing my father gives her age at the time of abuse at "3 or 4 or 5."[2] The above letters describe Lillian at ages six to eleven, from second through sixth grades. That being the case, the Conleys' friendship with Lillian began only one to three years after the alleged abuse had occurred. Yet they remember her as the beautiful, happy, delightful child we all knew.

Skeletons Without Bones

Regarding those same years, Lillian describes herself as always dirty, neglected, reclusive and, with Joy as the one glaring exception, without friends, and without social skills or contacts. She claims she was frightened of all people, most particularly her father, and that she was destructive and mutilating to herself. She remembers spending hours in seclusion, hiding under a table, or often up in our attic—masturbating.

Really? Our dark, unheated, unfinished attic that was bitterly cold in the New York winters and unbearably hot in the summers? I lived with her all those years, as did the rest of the family, and we never glimpsed the child she portrays. Now the added testimony of the Conleys exposes her memories as the fabrications they were. They never saw evidence of self-mutilation, or deviance from the characteristics and behavior of a typical happy, well-adjusted child. Further, they harbored no reservations about allowing their only daughter to spend countless hours in our home, including overnight and extended visits.

Louise has long been the family chronicler, delighting us on special occasions with her well-penned sentiments. One memoir most likely celebrates one of Lillian's birthdays:

> *Lillian Mae, my sister, born in 1942 a day or two prior to Thanksgiving at Fisher's home in the country up the road from New Hope Church and parsonage. Donna, age two, stayed with a family in the other direction. When we went to see Donna, she wanted to come home. Since there was no school Thursday or Friday, we brought her back with us.*
>
> *Lillian came home, the most beautiful baby doll, and Mom was proud of baby number seven as we all were. I remember the beautiful long dark hair Mom didn't want to cover up with a bonnet! She was welcomed as if to a King's house, and surely there was plenty of room for her!*[3]

The McGraw family moved to Miltonvale, Kansas for one year. Professor Knapp at Miltonvale Wesleyan College, a pho-

tographer by hobby, came to our house—a big, roomy mansion rented from the Phelps—and took pictures of Lillian in the rocker chair holding a doll, but most prized was her looking into a mirror with her pretty curls showing, as well as her face in the mirror. No one realized poor Donna Faye was crying because she didn't get her picture taken....

We had darling pictures of Donna and Lillian together and both were precious sweet darlings. After three years at Miltonvale Wesleyan High School, I went to Houghton, New York for my last year. On occasional weekends and during the summer I came home to Baldwinsville where we lived. I shared a small bedroom with Lillian and I remember how she would hug me when she went to sleep. I remember her and Roger in the wagon playing in the yard. I remember entering her photograph in a contest in Syracuse and being so sure she would win. I guess she didn't but we couldn't understand as she was definitely the most prettiest girl there ever was, with a precious smile and winning ways, curls, etc. We thought she was too little to walk the six blocks to school.... She was flower girl in my wedding...

Before Tim was born I had....to stay in bed most of the time. Lillian came the last two months to live with us and help me. She went to Junior High on Maple Street and we thought she was the greatest in the home and church and school. During that time the folks moved from Syracuse to Deanton, leaving Eddie in Syracuse (until that fall).

I recall how it upset Lillian when we got my birthday card from Daddy and it contained the sentence: "We had to leave Eddie. Alice would not let him come to Indiana with us."

We were sure that was the reason our Quiz Team, which Lillian was on, did not win the next evening, although she probably carried more than her weight and did her best for sure.

We had to leave her in Indiana in August. Mom was pregnant with Terry Lee....

The summer Lillian finished high school she tutored Millie in a college course so Millie could graduate. Millie paid tuition so Lillian could get credit for her time in class too. Lillian was in weddings for Millie, Lottie and Donna.

Lillian came to Missouri to live with us at Scott City and to attend Southeast Missouri College at Cape Girardeau, as well as to work in Southeast Missouri Hospital.

Then we up and moved to St. Louis to take the Wesleyan Chapel pastorate. It was an unplanned move, made before conference at the request of the Board. That left Lillian without us in Scott City.

Unfortunately, my husband and I did not realize how hard it was for her during that time of limited finances, time constraints, and a heavy work load—with no family close by. We were proud when Lillian could come to see us at St. Louis, and when she came in the spring or summer to stay and go to college in St. Louis.

Then she and Randall were dating which made us very, very proud, even though my husband's sister tried to warn Lillian that lots of girls wanted to go with Randall but he did not care for girls. She was surprised he did care so much for Lillian, finally.

Lillian had strep throat and fever around Thanksgiving time. I don't think Lillian really got over all the effects by the time of her wedding in February in Clay Center. She was still having diarrhea and was afraid what would happen in her wedding gown.

Trapped in the Trappings

We were thrilled Mom, Dad and kids could come for the wedding—with new clothes! They had just moved to Oklahoma from Indiana the month before. Daddy preached at Clay Center church that Sunday morning.

We still always felt like Lillian was the bestest with the mostest. As a nurses' aid, in college subjects, at home, with Sunday School class, singing and helping in children and youth activities, giving devotions at conference and camp, or whatever. Somehow everything was done with perfection. Not stereo-type perfection, but personalized into a new and much-appreciated beyond-perfection! And with more gracefulness or glamour than the way Millie and Donna did their own personalized presentations![4]

So we enjoyed Randall and Lillian being next door in St. Louis. Our boys really liked being with Randall. We overlooked Lillian's being busy and seeming withdrawn at times, burdened with work or school work and physical weakness. There were some disappointing situations [for her] in working at Barnes Hospital and later at Shriners' Crippled Childrens Hospital.

I can only regret from my depths if, in our appreciation and adulation of Lillian's abilities, we expected too much or if she felt we expected too much, and if we were part of the problem we did not dream existed, rather than being an answer.

Whatever that may have been, we still love Lillian, appreciate her, and know she will always come out on top and be used of God in HIS way, and rest in His will, and feel within that contentment and peace she always seemed to have!

God's faithfulness certainly reaches beyond man's misunderstandings. His rest is worth surrendering to and receiving! And will be perfected in Lillian, Randall and Cheree.

[Signed] Louise.

Skeletons Without Bones

Returning from Missouri to enter her sophomore year of high school at Deanton, Indiana, Lillian graduated at the head of her class three years later. These were the years Mitchell Scott, with his wife Angela at his side, pastored the church we attended. The letter they contributed regarding those years was addressed to me.

It was so good to hear from you and catch up on the Lord's on-going work in your family. We have lots of happy memories of your teenage years when we were your pastor at Deanton, Indiana.

You asked as to our perception of the McGraw family. We felt it was a real honor to have them move into our city and become a part of our church—all the way from Syracuse, New York. There was a specialness and love which radiated from your parents. They had enough for family and always seemed to have room for one more. Perhaps that is the reason your parents were the ones we left our first born, Mark, with for two and one half weeks while we went to Haiti. Mark so adapted himself to your household that he wasn't sure if he wanted to stay with your Mom and Dad when we returned, or go home with us. This made us a little jealous but it was not easy to compete with the McGraws.

When your family resources got thin, we talked about what we could afford to give them for a temporary boost. We thought fifty dollars was a pretty big amount out of our preacher's salary. But before we made out the check, we read a Scripture which said, "When your brother has a need, give him as much as he needs." We stretched our fifty dollars to one hundred dollars.

We experienced five years of revival while at Deanton. Even though your father was a seasoned teacher and student of the Word, he endeared himself to us by always "backing up" the preacher and the truth as revealed to us. Since we were realizing life-changing realities, it must have stretched Father McGraw a bit.

Lillian was clearly the favorite baby-sitter for our children. Her soft, gentle spirit made us comfortable whenever she came to our house. She was so original and able to come to their level. It made it easier for us to keep the schedule of the Word, prayer and church activity to which the Lord had called us in those days. We will never cease to be thankful for her lovely care of our children and becoming a dear friend to our family.

Our lives were further bonded with your family when the Lord prompted us to pray for the baby who had a serious affliction. The healing has been one which has stimulated our faith to pray and expect miracles for others.

We know the generational seed of this family will be reaping throughout unborn generations until Jesus comes. "The seed of the righteous shall be mighty upon the earth."

In our journey to the city we are happy to have been "a pilgrim and a stranger" with the McGraw family—"heirs of the same promise." "We thank God upon every remembrance of you."

[Signed] Lovingly, The Scotts.

It is plain that Lillian's current perception of herself and her family during her young years does not square with that of those who knew her best.

A letter addressed to Lillian from Vicki of "Sunday dinner pork chop" fame, also illustrates that fact.

Have been thinking about you often lately and should have written sooner. How are you doing? I got to see photos of ev-

eryone at the McGraw reunion.... Everyone looked wonderful and what memories it brought back!

Remember the good times you, Donna and I used to have? And when she wasn't around it was you and me. I remember people at church expressing confusion because they assumed Donna and I had the friendship, not realizing you and I were just as close and enjoyed a few years as buddies, comrades and dear, dear friends.

Some of my sweetest memories are of the two and three of us and me practically living in your home and being so readily accepted by a wonderful Christian family. Those years are among the best of my life.

I was thinking the two of us evidently were good for each other. You blessed my life in a never-to-be-forgotten manner. I loved you, Lilly, you and Donna, and our relationship. I love you across the miles. Thank you for all you gave to, shared with, and left to me on parting.

God bless you. Stay well and happy.
[Signed] Love, Vicki.

Does this letter portray Lillian as a malfunctioning social misfit? Not by a long shot! Vicki's own words to me over the phone were, "I hope you won't be offended, Donna. But when you left for college, Lillian stepped into your shoes and I hardly knew the difference."

Am I offended by her words? Certainly not. Neither am I surprised. For we were three good friends, sharing each other's companionship, possessions and secrets. We even shared friendships with the same boys, sometimes going places together as a group, sometimes going on single or double dates. This continued over a period of a couple of years without a single instance of the wrangling and jealousies that are normally the consequence of that type of shared relationships.

Perhaps the most telling testimony of her mental and emotional stability comes from the pen of sixteen-year-old Lillian herself. In a letter postmarked Deanton, Indiana, addressed to Louise dated April 14, 1958, Lillian wrote:

Dear Louise and family,

You've probably about forgotten who I am. It's been so long since I've written.

We've been real busy here. Revival for the past two weeks ended yesterday. Evangelists were Carrie Hazzard and Lois Richardson. They are really good! Do you know them or anything? They had morning services which Mother went to every morning with Terry and Eddie. Except three mornings Peggy or Donna stayed with the boys.

The baby [Terry Lee] is six weeks old tonight. He cried day and night almost constantly the first three weeks home. We all thought we'd go nuts.

Mom's been feeling pretty good. Was quite tired the first two or three weeks home. She's feeling okay now except when he cries. **I think it bothers her more to hear him cry than any other of her babies. She holds him a lot when he cries, gives him a pacifier, sometimes feeds him his milk early and she has even given him cereal a few times.** *[Emphasis mine.]*

Terry's real cute. Looks quite a bit like Timmie did. His once black hair is not so black. Will probably get real light because his eyebrows and eye lashes are. He eats good. Six ounces every four hours of Simalac liquid, except when Mom gives in and feeds him early. He laughs when talked to and likes to be held. He learned that when he had (and sometimes

> still has) colic. The church ladies had a shower for him. He got lots of diapers, suits, etc. He has lots of second hand clothes too.
>
> Daddy's prouder'n a peacock over him, too. Had Mom take him to the Publishing House [where Dad worked] two weeks ago.
>
> Has Millie told you of her plans? Well, this isn't positive yet, we're sort of planning this: to come to get Millie after school's out. Mom, Daddy, Donna, Eddie, Terry and I will come. We'll go to Madison and Washington (maybe), Wichita, Enid, Alva and Jamestown. That way you could all see Terry Lee. Millie said she'd pay for the trip because if she came on the train or bus it would be $30 or something. We're planning. Not yet sure but I thought I'd tell you anyhow.
>
> Scotts ask about you often. We sure like the church here!

She continues to write a few paragraphs about what is happening at church among the teenagers. Then in a more personal vein she says:

> The Lord means a lot to me. He's really near all the time. I'm reading the Bible through and am in II Kings. I really enjoy the Old Testament, too.
>
> I don't know if I've ever thanked you for putting up with me last spring and summer. I really enjoyed my stay there and that's where I came to know Christ personally. Tell everybody there thanks for the help they gave me...
>
> I suppose you knew we kept Starr while Scotts were in Haiti? We had her three weeks. She was about fourteen or fifteen months then.[5]

Trapped in the Trappings

> Eddie's happy here and is a little scamp. Sometimes Mom says that he just starts crying and says, "Why did you pack my clothes and let Alice take me?"
>
> When he saw the picture of me and your boys, he said, "That's Terry and Lilly but who's that little boy?"
>
> Write soon if you have a chance. Tell Etta it's her turn and I'm going to try to write Faith. Pray for us. Love always.
> [Signed] Your little sister, Lillian.

She adds three P.S.'s which include the following statements:

> How is everybody there? I'd like to see them all again. Maybe I will! I have a picture of Larkie. Faith wanted me to have one of her too but I didn't get it.

In this letter Lillian herself verifies her happy home life, putting the lie to her own later version of it. She writes as a teenager who loves and is loved by her family. She describes Mother taking care of Terry Lee, and she reveals her own interest in the details of his care, even to naming his formula.

In referring to the previous summer when she had eagerly assisted Louise at the birth of her third son, it is clear Lillian had made several friends with whom she exchanged pictures and correspondence.

Was our little sister reclusive? Anti-social? Friendless? An unloved Cinderella forced into servitude, dutifully tending babies because no one else would? Only a pseudo psychologist with a hidden agenda could come to such a conclusion!

I noted with interest the use of the nickname "Lilly" in two of the letters.

Dr. French had explained to us that Lillian's abuse had been so extreme that she had split into two personalities, Lillian and Lilly. He said as a child Lillian had rejected her nickname, for "Lilly" had become the name of the alter-ego. "Lilly" was the one that bore the brunt and the marks of mistreatment. "Lillian," on the other hand, was the host or dominant personality, who had to cope with her miserable life of doing all the housework and baby-tending in our dysfunctional household. "Lillian" struggled to keep "Lilly" submerged in the Limbo of her forgotten past. That is, until Dr. French identified and exposed the spurned "Lilly" and integrated the warring entities into one struggling personality.

An elaborately-contrived fairy tale, illustrative of a therapist's creativity that often passes for intelligence. But it contains not a trace of truth.

The entire theory is negated by two of the above letters. Vicki addresses Lillian by the nickname "Lilly," which indicates its usage was alive and well during Lillian's late teenage years. Even more revealing, in her letter to Louise, Lillian herself quoted her younger brother as calling her "Lilly," showing that Lillian accepted the use of that name for herself at age sixteen.

No, in spite of Dr. French's damnable theorizing, there never existed two personalities of Lillian. No indication exists that "Lilly" was either a repressed personality or a rejected name. Lilly was simply a nickname, one and the same person as Lillian, who lived and flourished in her father's house. She left her father's house a whole, integrated, functioning young person, eager to fulfil her dreams—her *own* dreams—of becoming a missionary doctor after the order of her idol, Dr. Marilyn Birch.

How does one explain, then, the broken, tortured Lillian of her early adult years?

I admit I don't really know for certain. I never saw that Lillian. I was miles away when she bit and mutilated her body, or when she lived on the edge of suicide, or when she screamed for long periods of time and was generally a non-productive, malfunctioning piece of humanity, living under the illusion her father had raped her and her husband was trying to kill her.

I do not know all that happened between the time she left home to attend college in New York State in 1961 and when she arrived on the West Coast a decade or so later. But I *do* know for certain what my sister was like before she left home, and I *do* know, without question and without re-interpretation from an outsider, what our home was like.

Starting with what I already know, I can do what Dr. French did—I can reconstruct her past. Only I will do a better job because I will use first-hand knowledge and verifiable facts gathered from witnesses of the events in question.

As a high school senior, Lillian was functioning as an intelligent, well-balanced teenager, enjoying good relationships with her family and her friends. Her skills for dealing with children of all ages were legendary and much sought-after by mothers on the lookout for reliable baby sitters. After her graduation, Lillian continued living at home while commuting to classes at a nearby liberal arts college for her freshman year of college.

During Lillian's last year of high school and her first year of college, she spent a great deal of time with a young lady who had recently come to live in our home and who had become to us "sister number eight." A recent college graduate, Lottie stood on the threshold of a teaching career. Coming to us as a house guest of my sister Millie, Lottie found in Mother a sympathetic audience who listened to her stories of a troubled past. "House guest" metamorphosed to resident, and Lottie lived with us until her marriage in 1962.

Lottie told us of repeated sexual abuse by her older brother. She implicated not only her brother, but her mother and other brothers and sisters as party to her exploitation. She insisted they all were aware of the incestual relationship but refused to acknowledge its existence, or intervene on Lottie's behalf.

If you, the reader, are thinking that all this has a remarkably familiar ring, you are miles ahead of my sister's high-priced psychologist. One has to wonder why, in digging around in Lillian's past, he failed to discover that Lillian spent untold hours, many sessions lasting far into the night, soaking up the morbid details of Lottie's violation by her brother.

All the feelings and emotions suffered by Lottie were rehashed over and over again to the attentive ears and fertile mind of my young sister.

Skeletons Without Bones

Lillian has told me several times over that she sees ideas and concepts in *vivid, detailed mental pictures—to a degree not experienced by other people.*

How anyone has the ability to compare the intensity and quality of her own mental images with everyone else's alludes me. However that may be, it is inevitable that Lillian, while listening to Lottie's detailed descriptions, would have vicariously experienced an incestual relationship, with all its attending emotional trauma. *Once visualized, these events would remain forever indelibly recorded in Lillian's memory, malleable material for future manipulation by an opportunistic expert hypnotist.*

For her second year of college Lillian transferred to Houghton College in New York State to pursue what she felt to be her calling—medical missions.

At Houghton, Lillian found herself needing to excel in a highly competitive collegiate environment, hundreds of miles from home, without the support of family and friends to which she was accustomed. No small town church nurtured her, no dearly loved pastor and wife stood ready to assist her over the rough places. No big, boisterous family, no Mom and Dad stood by providing emotional stability. No little brothers and sisters needed her time or vied for her attention. Not even a big, crowded dormitory teeming with girls helped fill the voids, for she rented a single-occupant room upstairs in the home of two sedate elderly sisters, the Misses Fancher.

Without customary distractions, it is not difficult to imagine that Lillian, accustomed to being Number One academically, would throw herself whole-heartedly into maintaining that position. But now she competed, not in a small midwestern high school, but in the big leagues, pitted against the cream of the crop in a prestigious private college in Western New York State.

So how does one excel in such an aggressive, intellectual arena? By Lillian's own admission, she used the common crutches found on any drugstore shelf.

No doubt she intended to use them carefully and sparingly— just until this paper was finished, until that collateral was read, until another deadline was met and one more important test was aced. "Uppers" allowed study far into the night, "downers" induced sleep for the few remaining hours. Once the cycle is begun, how does one break loose?

Some people may be fortunate enough to suffer no lasting damage from such a regimen. Others do not fare so well. In a family with identified cases of drug-sensitivity,[6] it is reasonable to assume that Lillian's crutches turned out to be her undoing, especially when coupled with her failure to offset her drug consumption with even a minimal amount of nourishing food. I know this is fact, for when Gary and I visited her at Thanksgiving time, she confessed to us that her landladies constantly fussed at her for not eating.

Persons who regularly counsel drug users tell me that a person's memory can be adversely affected by misuse of medications, whether in the form of illegal drugs, prescribed medication or over-the-counter varieties.

It follows that Lillian could have suffered drastic personality changes, including nervousness, mood swings and depression. Her obsession with making superior grades, while losing ground physically, mentally and emotionally, would exacerbate the downward spiral. Living alone, her only contacts total strangers—who would have detected the difference?

Although she didn't return to Houghton College in New York State, Lillian did continue her education the next several years in Missouri.

At this point I must begin to speculate, for by this time I had married and my contacts with Lillian were minimal. Did she continue use of chemical crutches, coupled with her poor nutritional practices? By all indications, she did. In addition, she got married and bore a child, adding new demands to her already depleted reserves as she continued to work as well as pursue a degree.

Although I saw Lillian only at an occasional holiday gathering during the next few years, one of our younger brothers offered some insight which he contributed to our *Document of Defense* collection.

Skeletons Without Bones

May 1993 - From John [and Marcia]

My point in saying what went on is not to hurt anyone in the family regardless of anyone's opinions. The very people we are talking about are people I love and care about. Each one played an important part in my life.

Lillian helped me when I was small in school and in college, too. Randall opened his home to me so I could go to college. Earlier, Ginny and Lyle took me in and treated me as their own and gave me a new lease on life—not only in school skills, but more importantly in my abilities to succeed in normal living. Lyle probably gave me the greatest gift of all—the gift of believing in myself enough to be myself—a square peg in a round-hole world.

It only took Marcia a short while after she moved to Oklahoma City to realize that Lillian was truly sick. Lillian went to a Dr. Luckey (spelling?) frequently for care and took lots of medication. A few times she went over to his house in the evening and spent several hours alone with him. We never knew what went on there, but we knew a doctor/patient relationship like that was out of line.

Lillian managed to keep the house functioning with a cleaning lady and frequent meals brought in by Randall. Cheree wasn't neglected, but Lillian was very busy with school and being sick. I wish I had known what a burden I probably was for them at that time. I probably shouldn't have stayed with them.

The thing I noticed most was Lillian digging at her face and making sores and making every incidence in her life somehow be based on sex. She controlled all of our lives by getting "sick" whenever faced with something disagreeable to her.

I felt like all of this was extremely hard on Randall. I knew that the constant chatter about sex, including all the male workers at school who supposedly made sexual advances to her constantly, bothered him. I know for a fact there was rare sex at home despite all the talk.

When they decided to move to Washington, Dr. Luckey thought that was wonderful because he knew of Dr. French's reputation and agreed with his philosophy—which is Freudian psychology—that teaches sex is your problem and your parents cause your sexual problems. (This statement is mine-MJM.)

This is the end of our knowledge of them and their problems. We don't say any of this to gossip and would never have said any of this except in defense of our parents. When Lillian brought up the fact that Daddy had raped her, I wasn't shocked because I knew she was not of sound mind. But it did infuriate me because I know Dad so well and had spent so much time talking man to man. The girls only knew him as a great man—as a minister.

I feel the time has come when this family has to come together on this issue in a consensus or we will lose the very spirit Daddy created over a delusion of a sick person whose mind had been polluted by a convicted pervert who has little time left in this world....

After Lillian revealed the dirty deed, [Randall's sister] came for a visit and we talked with her about this. At the time she was a social worker at a prison in Kansas and dealt specifically with sexual deviants in the prison system. She was writing a chapter for a textbook on the subject during that time and she stated that she did not believe the tale that had been told. There is a definite pattern a man of this caliber follows. The man starts abusing the oldest girl first and discards her as she matures in order to use the next in line and so on down the line of girls in the family. The fact that Lillian is the only one with this memory is totally contrary to professionals in the field.

Rose, you want happy memories. The most precious memory of Dad is one I talked about at the reunion and one he never knew about. That is why it is so precious because it was my true blue Dad and the basis for my faith and definitely worth putting in print.

When I was a little guy, before I became a Christian, I always knew when I heard noises in the dark, it wasn't the bogeyman— it was Dad. In the wintertime, when I would still be in bed, I could look out in the living room and see Dad praying, mumbling—not words I could understand. I knew that if I kept staring into the dark, I would finally hear the furnace click on and it would light in a yellow ball. Then I would see the stick figure leaning over a chair with his knees on a pillow. Even as a boy, I knew what I was seeing was not fake, it was real. It gave me a peace and security and made me wish for the same in my life.

Years later, when I was already married and we were moving Mom to Texas, I found that pillow and if you looked carefully, you could see where Dad's bony knees had worn it thin from kneeling on it.

After coming back from Washington at age thirteen and after traveling to St. Louis to see Louise, the folks decided we would go see Uncle Kenneth and Aunt Reba. Dad was never known for his driving ability and if you had any doubts about a true and living God, they would soon be squelched after riding with Dad. We were driving at night, which was an added hazard, and it was real foggy (saints preserve us!) We crossed a railroad track and Dad said, "Do you hear that?" and we did.

Trapped in the Trappings

Dad moved on and the train noise got louder, but we couldn't see anything. Finally Dad just stopped and said, "We can't go any farther because I don't know where this thing is."

We no more than got stopped than the train roared by right in front of us—we were just shy of the new tracks. It was an extremely frightening experience that Dad could not have dealt with on his own.

Dad used to love to kid with Mom. He always had paper in hand so he would use it as a weapon. He made paper torpedoes (big bunches of paper) and when Mom would bend over, he would lob them at her keister. She would look up and say, "Daddy!" in an exasperated tone and he would pretend he didn't know what she was getting after him for. Sometimes she would throw them back and try to get him.

Dad could make the best puddings and pies. If you would get up early enough on Saturday, he would fix vanilla or chocolate pudding, whichever you wanted. He would get up and go to the kitchen to make a pie and his pumpkin, cherry and apple pies were great. He cleaned up after himself, too.

As for this new revelation from Lillian. Now that Dad has become old news, Mom is her target for physical abuse. We were all spanked, but not abused. No one was ever abused when Mom or Dad was home with us. With all the children in one home, of course there needed to be discipline. In all the time I was growing up, I never saw anyone whip Lillian ever, but I did hear her get scolded by Mom's tongue for wrongdoing. If Mom's iron hand was going to come down on somebody, it came down on the boys, not the girls. We most generally got just what we deserved. I realize that with today's "enlightened" standards, it would be considered abuse since these days children should not be disciplined at all.

As far as I remember, Lillian worked so hard to please everyone and for her not to succeed would have been rare because she was the "little princess." By the way, she made great fudge!

When Mom has served her purpose, who will be the next abuser in the family!

[Signed] JEM

A note from Marcia—Being raised in a non-Christian home, I can see the gift God gave all of you children so much more easily. I would have been blessed if I had Christian parents to lead by example. I feel blessed to have married a man with his great heritage. Don't let the Devil destroy the heritage—pass it on to the next generation and beyond!

To summarize, Lillian was prescribed medication during her young teen years to diminish her menstrual discomfort. She used chemical substances to help her get through her second year of college. Five or six years later we have John's witness that she "took lots of medication." Still later, under Dr. French's care, medications were used in conjunction with her therapy. These facts indicate a possible case of chemical dependency encompassing Lillian's entire youth and young adulthood.

However innocently it may have developed, I submit that chemical dependency explains Lillian's disintegrated, non-functional personality observed by some of my siblings and their families. In the above-mentioned condition, Lillian presented herself first to Dr. Luckey in Oklahoma City and later to Dr. French in Washington State. I believe that instead of helping her recover, they took advantage of her unstable physical, mental and emotional condition.

These two Freudian counselors fostered in Lillian an additional dependency on themselves with their false diagnoses and bogus therapies. Filling her mind with heresies, they assisted her in creating false memories—memories which have many of the same components as the accounts of sexual abuse she heard from Lottie.

I argue that those years of drug dependency left Lillian unable to distinguish between her own past, and that which she experienced vicariously through her visualization of Lottie's past.

At least one of her therapists—namely, Dr. French—was himself an unscrupulous practitioner, knowingly and purposely preying upon his clients to his own financial and egocentric gain, all the while gratifying a seemingly insatiable lust for sex and power.

I fear that my sister has invested so much of her life, herself and her identity in her "survivorship" that she dares not consider a different conclusion. I believe she knows her house of cards could not withstand an onslaught of facts and logic.

Therefore she remains today trapped in the trappings, inveigled in the investments that had promised to set her free.

The Lillian that people see today is the "survivor." She has crawled out of her shell. She is physically well and attractive. She relates, socializes and rolls with life's punches. For several years she has kept a demanding schedule as she raises her autistic grandson Heath. She takes him to multiple therapy-related appointments, and maintains a rigorous regimen that has produced unusual improvement for Heath.

The credit for Heath's achievements goes to my sister Lillian and her unflagging efforts on his behalf. I respect and admire Lillian's success in the face of seemingly insurmountable odds.

I believe these attributes reveal the real Lillian, the adult version of the gentle sister who shared my childhood. Her accomplishments with Heath may also be the fulfillment of her childhood dreams.

No, there is no impressive medical degree behind her name. But no lettered professional could have brought about the degree of progress she has helped Heath to achieve by setting aside her personal goals and dedicating herself with missionary-like zeal on his behalf.

Did someone force her to do it? Of course not! Something deep within her constrained her, motivating her to make the choices she has made. Could it be the out-cropping of those early desires and motives that led her as a young child to desire to be a medical missionary "like Dr. Marilyn Birch?"

The burden Lillian carries stands between herself and those who love her, for they recognize it for what it is—a lie that has nearly destroyed her and that has tortured her entire family.

She could right these wrongs by assuming responsibility, renouncing her heresies and setting the record straight. In so doing she would find complete forgiveness, wholeness and peace she cannot now imagine.

Would it be difficult for her to do? No doubt—at first. But not as difficult as holding together a house of cards while dwelling within its flimsy shelter. I pray she will soon put her past behind her, forgiven and forgotten, and embrace and enjoy her real past, her present and her future.

The Lord has promised more than survivorship. He has promised to make us more than conquerors, predicated only on finding and embracing the truth. Somewhere in her heart of hearts, I believe Lillian knows the truth. I believe she knows there was no abuse, and there was no incest. She should also know she was welcomed, cuddled and fussed over. Her father and mother loved, nurtured and protected her.

If her over-medicated years have eradicated her history, she is fortunate to be "surrounded by so great a crowd of witnesses" who would gladly reconstruct it for her—without the influence of hypnosis, drugs, leaky psychological theories, or unrestrained lust.

One big family waits, anxious to welcome her back!

CHAPTER NINETEEN

Beware! Epidemic!

When Lillian and my three nieces rejected our written defense of my father, it left me emotionally depleted regarding the whole subject. The hope that, in the end, reason and logic would prevail had dissipated. I could not comprehend how Lillian and Ginny and their families could retain their devotion to Dr. French in the face of his well-documented scandal, when they had so easily spurned our father on an indefensible trumped-up charge.

In February of 1994 my husband Gary and I attended a local meeting of supporters of the *False Memory Syndrome Foundation (FMSF)*[1].

Pain pervaded the room filled with one hundred and twenty people who were trudging the same mucky road we know so well. Most of the attenders had had their worlds flipped upside down, with traumatic court trials scarring their recent pasts or looming in their near futures. Victims of a system run amuck, their horror stories could rival anything being portrayed on daytime soap operas.

To my surprise, I learned that day that our family had emerged as one of the more fortunate ones. No lawsuit resulted in loss of property and lifelong savings. Daddy had not languished in a prison cell. The tragedy of Alzheimer's disease may have served as God's vehicle to fulfill His promise that "*all things work together for good to them that love God*" (Romans 8:28, King James Version), shielding him from full comprehension of his plight.

The couple seated next to me grieved the loss of a son. After entering therapy, he had cut off all contact with them. Confused and broken, when a call came from his therapist asking them to meet with their son in his office, their hopes skyrocketed. A breakthrough! Oh, happy day! They could scarcely wait!

They hadn't a clue! They had considered every possibility but this one. Their mistake, as was mine, was that they reckoned within the bounds of reality. No one told them their enemy cares nothing for reality, logic, history, or science. They had been ushered into an unreal world where fantasy reigns!

They had gone to the therapist's office full of hope, only to be clobbered with charges of sexual abuse. I couldn't help but recall that scene some years earlier in Terry, Montana, when Lillian had said to me, "I wish I could tell Mother," and I had vowed to myself, "You will never do to Mother what you did to me!"

Fourteen years later in Seattle, Washington, the haggard faces and stooped shoulders of the prematurely old couple seated beside us confirmed to us we had made the right decision. We have since discovered it is a frequent practice of some therapists to take family members, one by one, into the inner sanctum to brainwash them, destroy them, and/or intimidate them into silence.

Not all the attendees of that meeting were victims of recovered repressed memories. We talked to parents whose minor children had been snatched from them by over-reaching authorities. One father told us his kindergarten daughter had been taught at school about "bad touching." Afterward, the children were grilled. "Has anyone ever touched you that way?" They were encouraged to think about it and were pressed for answers. The method sounds strikingly similar to Dr. French's "intensive."

Eager to comply, this man's six-year-old daughter suggested her father may have touched her private parts.

Beware! Epidemic!

As a vulture tears into carrion, the teacher jumped on that one with talons extended. How did it happen? Where was she?

"My daddy gave me a bath."

Teacher: "How long ago?"

"I think when I was three."

Anyone not totally brain dead knows you cannot give a child a decent bath without washing the genital area. But the brain dead are not all confined to intensive care units.

That little girl never returned to her home. *Child Protective Services* paid a visit to the family and left with the other children in tow, crying hysterically, including the two-year-old they pulled from the protesting mother's arms. At this writing the parents have been childless for two years.

At the trial the father was promised the children would be returned if he would just admit his guilt and subject himself to counseling. Sounds like a simple enough solution. One slight problem: he had sworn to tell the truth. The truth is, he was not guilty of molesting his daughter. So the children are growing up deprived of their parents. The man and his wife spend all their resources seeking to regain custody of their children.

I am humbled at the man's courage to refuse to "play along" with the system. Perhaps he knows that other men who have succumbed to offers of leniency in exchange for a confession are serving time. They discovered too late that:

- When sexual abuse is the charge, the rules suddenly change. Authorities consider the accused "guilty until proven innocent."
- Authorities will promise almost anything in order to extract a confession, because:

    1. Authorities feel no obligation to keep promises made to an accused child molester.
    2. An unsubstantiated accusation puts a man through hell. A confession, however it may be extruded, seals his fate there forever.

The majority of those attending that meeting of FMSF supporters, however, had been accused of sexual abuse as a result of recovered repressed memories. As we compared notes, I discovered that my account of our family's experience brought near despair to my listeners. For many of the families, it was a nightmare just begun. For others the horror was of three, four, maybe five years' duration. They hoped it would soon end. When they found out ours began over fourteen years ago, they did not want to even contemplate such a possibility.

Their next question inevitably was, "Is your father still living?"

When I said, "No," near panic set in. Tears welled up as they admitted, "Our worst nightmare is that we will die without our name being cleared, still alienated from our children and grandchildren."

I ceased telling my story. If I could not give them hope, at least I would not deepen their despair.

The highlight of the day came when a young lady called Sarah gave testimony that did bring hope to every person there. She stood before us, a real, live retractor—the first most of us had ever met. She personified for each of us a lost daughter or sister.

Only six weeks into her return to reality, Sarah was also glimpsing for the first time the "other side." She had come to the meeting incognito, not sure she was ready for identification and exposure. But as the meeting progressed, her reticence turned to eagerness and she consented to speak to us and answer our questions.

Instantly we loved her. Never had a speaker faced a more eager, a more supportive audience. Poised and articulate, she told us what we longed to hear. Her story was so familiar to us that we could have told much of it ourselves. But she told it from the inside.

She spoke of her intense fixation on her therapist. The total trust in the integrity and knowledge of the counselor, augmented by drugs and hypnosis—all the usual components were present, relentlessly pushing her toward the horrible discovery of what had happened to her at the hands of her family. Reading assignments and testimonials by other "survivors" added momentum, propelling her toward her counsellor's predetermined goal.

Perhaps the most insidious stratagem used by therapists is that of taking innocent events of the client's life and re-interpreting them to fit the therapist's warped presuppositions.[2] I'll never forget Sarah's words:

> *My therapist turned the members of my family into monsters before my very eyes, the way she reinterpreted for me everything they did and everything they said. She made them all into monsters.*

The anger of the audience was almost tangible as parents remembered the sacrifices they gladly made to pay the lucrative fees that had enabled some shrink to make monsters of them!

You need not tell me her story and ours are exceptions to the rule! Over twenty thousand families in the United States and two thousand families in Canada have contacted the *False Memory Syndrome Foundation* with similar accounts during its first five and one-half years of existence. Surveys reveal that for every household, fifty to seventy individuals are significantly affected, bringing the total to over 1,000,000 Americans, and over 100,000 Canadians who have gone through what we have suffered. And for every family that has contacted the Foundation, many more remain unidentified.

We are not talking about a few isolated cases. We are talking near epidemic proportions! We're speaking of a communicable disease, deliberately spawned and transmitted from mind to mind in virulent incubators known as therapists' offices.

The good news is that it is a totally preventable disease. The public can be immunized by being made aware of the danger that lurks in contaminated areas and by avoiding prolonged contact with infected persons masquerading as counselors or "survivors."

Perhaps the saddest cases are those in which confessions have been extracted from accused fathers under pressure exerted by heavy-handed professionals. I experienced some of the self-doubt and mental confusion which results from an unexpected accusation. This mental terror and turmoil must be greatly multiplied when a person finds that he himself stands accused. I understand the pressure under which some fathers succumb to falsely admitting guilt in hopes of bringing closure to the chaos thrust upon them and their families.

Through brainwashing techniques and outright lies, these men are often led to believe that it is possible—in fact, it is almost certain—that they are unable to remember their own crimes against their children because they, like their daughters, have repressed the memories. Once an accused father buys into the Pandora's box of repressed memories, he finds it far less painful to entertain the possibility of lapses in his own moral integrity than to doubt the veracity or the sanity of his own beloved daughter.

This is more easily comprehended if one remembers that fathers—correctly lauded as heros—do not hesitate to put their lives on the line by jumping into raging waters or rushing into burning buildings to save the life of one of their offspring—even if the child's danger is a direct result of rebellion and/or disobedience. However, there are no hero's crowns for men who make desperate and preposterous confessions, sacrificing their own reputations and integrity in an effort to save the honor and reputation of a daughter in the throes of "recovered repressed memories."

Assured that their confession will resurrect memory from its burial site and will produce recall, men will capitulate simply because they have discovered it is totally futile to challenge the experts,[3] and they have been shamed into "sparing their innocent daughters further trauma and embarrassment."

No one warns the accused that, while emerging repressed memories are readily accepted as capricious entities—able to disappear and re-appear, ever changing and expanding under therapeutic scrutiny—this is never the case with confessions. No matter how heavy-handed the extraction method used, or how tenuously it is given, once a confession is made, it is cast in bronze, forever irretractable. The man is forever branded a pedophile—one who preyed upon his own children.

CHAPTER TWENTY

The Turning of the Tide

During the summer and fall of 1993, the trickle of media attention given to the subject of recovered repressed memories swelled to a steady stream.

The *False Memory Syndrome Foundation* deserves much of the credit for this increased visibility. Until this organization appeared on the scene, each family suffered the ravages of false accusations as an isolated unit, seeking to shield its accused from unwelcome exposure and additional pain and embarrassment. For over a decade my family, like many others, had no knowledge it had ever happened to anyone else. Journalists either did not know we existed, or were themselves too brainwashed or too intimidated to tackle the "therapeutic cartel."

But exposure has come—finally. Major periodicals feature articles on the subject. We see frequent national TV coverage via talk shows, and investigative programs exploring and publicizing the phenomenon. A landmark lawsuit in California and a highly publicized retraction in Chicago have increased general awareness and sympathy. "False memory" has become a household concept.

I have tried to buy every book and every article that has appeared on the market concerning this subject. As my collection expanded, I realized it contained no account of how a family dealt with the devastation of recovered false memories over the long haul. Neither did I find anything written from a Christian perspective, though I know several Christian families that have suffered through the experience.

When my son Dustin repeatedly reminded me that this was a story begging to be told, I refused to consider it. The task appeared too big, the story too painful, the climate too hostile, the outcome too costly.

But as 1993 drew to a close, the climate had turned from hostile to curious, if not sympathetic. People no longer considered it vulgar to suggest a therapist might not be infallible! My sisters and nieces may have been uninterested in hearing our story, but I felt the rest of the world stood poised to listen.

My current job generated little stress and my energy level had peaked to an all-time high. The empty status of my nest appeared to be permanent. Consequently, I began to feel challenged rather than overwhelmed by Dustin's idea of writing a book. A husband eager to lend support and assistance, and a niece standing by with pencil poised provided the final impetus that pushed me over the brink.

The project has proven itself a rewarding one. When Lillian's accusations had erupted, they left an ugly volcano of filth piled in the forefront of my memories, obscuring the scenery beyond.

Writing the manuscript has taken me back beyond the eruption and its devastation, revealing once again the beautiful terrain that had formed the backdrop and turf of my growing up years. Once again I could see my family as it had been before the accusations had defaced the landscape. Retracing my steps back to the present from that perspective, the blemish has lost its potency. It no longer dominates my horizon nor obliterates my true past.

But even as the book took shape and neared completion, unknown to me, another chapter was being written.

The Turning of the Tide

One weekend in July of 1994, Gary and I attended a family camp-out. Soon after our arrival, Ginny's daughter Danita excitedly showed me a book she and her sister Shannon had discovered.[1] The book's chapter headings were made up of concepts or character traits such as "Honesty," "Integrity," and "Obedience to and Honor of Parents." Each chapter then listed passages in the Bible which addressed that particular concept.

Both girls began studying the Scriptures indicated. While they were mastering the Word of God, the Word of God mastered them! Without consulting the other, each girl began to realize how far she had drifted from living according to Biblical principles. Though they had considered themselves Christians, lack of Scriptural foundation or comprehension left them without an anchor to prevent such a drift.

Always effervescent, Danita talked eagerly about her new-found insights. Caught up in her rendition, at first I failed to detect the direction her story was taking and the implications of it. Finally, somewhat stunned, I realized Danita was telling me that through her study, she had discovered that the concepts she had previously embraced were false. During the past two months she had grasped the extent of her deception and had categorically repudiated it in its totality.

Her sister Shannon, without collaborating with Danita, had reached the exact same conclusions! Their eyes now opened, they no longer believed what they had learned from Dr. French and their Aunt Lillian, including the accusations leveled against their grandfather.

I stood as one dazed. These two nieces, along with their sister Kim and my sister Lillian, were the ones to whom Anna and I had unsuccessfully presented our *Document of Defense*. The significance of these girls boldly stating their defection could scarcely be comprehended or overstated.

I marveled at Danita's insights and conclusions concerning her previous deception. She confessed that for the first time in her adult life, confusion had been replaced by a sense of peace.

Describing her experience to me, she commented, "After one domino fell, they all went." Her terminology reminded me of that of a complainant at Dr. French's hearing when I asked her what my role should be as I awaited my family's emergence from Dr. French's cult.

"They are desperately holding together their house of cards. When one card goes—and it will go—the whole structure will collapse. *Don't do anything, just be there for them.*"

Now, two years later, I was witnessing what I hoped was the prelude to the fulfillment of her prediction, expressed in a similar metaphor by my newly-enlightened niece. Would my sisters follow suit? I could not help but think the time was near. I even dared hope that by the time this book was ready for publication, the final chapter could be written by our own retractor.

One surprise that came out of Danita's about-face was her admission that our aborted effort to give our *Document of Defense* to Lillian helped to open the eyes of my nieces.

All their growing-up years, Danita and her sisters had heard Lillian recite the events of her horrible life, as she described herself as the mistreated little victim of the entire family. Only after years of therapy from Dr. French had she emerged brave and strong, finally able to stand up to her tormenters, equipped with strength that other people only dreamed of possessing.

My nieces had watched as Lillian slowly emerged from a cowering, fear-driven recluse to the daring, resolute crusader they perceived her to be, full of bravado and spiritual insights. Eagerly they soaked up all the wisdom they could from the heroic Dr. French and his protegé, their Aunt Lillian.

But the day we ventured to offer our *Document of Defense*, they witnessed the scene as Anna and I approached Lillian without being malicious or confrontational. They observed as we tried to reason with Lillian about her own contradictions. They saw her respond in anger, and then cower behind her timeworn mantra, "My family never did love me."

The girls had then jumped in to defend Lillian. But now Danita confessed to me that even as they did so, they had been confused

The Turning of the Tide

and angry. "What has happened to the brave and self-confident Lillian who had all the right answers and the wonderful reservoir of strength? Why is she cowering and whimpering, making it necessary for us to defend her as if she were a helpless child? Why can't she answer the questions her sisters are raising? And why is all the anger and meanness coming from *our side* rather than from Aunt Anna and Aunt Donna?"

Later, the three sisters—Danita, Shannon and Kim—often discussed and puzzled over the strange events of that afternoon when two of their unenlightened aunts came with a mission to visit their mentor—Aunt Lillian.

So I discovered that God, after all, had taken our failure, our "nothing," and, out of it, He fashioned something quite wonderful!

For the present, we have no retraction from our accusing sister. However, we do have a hard-hitting statement given by Danita in a letter she wrote to one of her brothers the summer of 1994.

I include Danita's observations to show her about-face after she renounced her infatuation with the maze of therapy; to show how diametrically at odds are the precepts of modern therapy with the plain teaching of Biblical Christianity; and to show how God was, after all, answering prayer concerning that which I had, just the summer before, all but given up on.

> *About a month ago I discovered I was so double-minded and backslidden that my Christianity was like a hideous joke.*
>
> *This discovery came in several steps. First, God impressed upon my heart that whom He disciplines (disciples), He loves. I began to sense that correction from God was a good thing, bestowed on his beloved children, not doled out at random.*
>
> *When I read the book* INSTRUCTION IN RIGHTEOUSNESS, *I became totally convicted by the section titled "Backslidden/ Double-Mindedness" (to name but one). I was ripe for correction. I mean, I welcomed it!*

For many years I have complained that I am miserable. I blamed everyone I could think of—my parents, God, friends, enemies and total strangers.

I "became a Christian" and immediately went out and sought therapy to get my life in order. I don't know what I thought God was for, but obviously something other than redemption—immediate redemption, at least.

I used to practically chant all the filthy blasphemous epithets I could think of and I scourged my children with obscenities. Now I don't. Not because I try not to. I was delivered from it.

If I could have received deliverance from therapy, I surely would have after ten years with a Ph.D. (i.e. "has all the answers") psychologist. If any of the bogus spirituality of the New Age could have healed me, it would have, because I dabbled in it. But I didn't find my help there. I found it in Jesus Christ.

In therapy, paying through the nose for the promise of "inner peace," I continually griped about feeling I had not had enough rest; I was always fatigued. I lamented over not producing any fruits of the Spirit: love, joy, peace, longsuffering, kindness, goodness, faithfulness, gentleness and self-control. Especially self-control. I complained that I always felt raunchy inside.

In therapy I blamed my parents for all that was lacking in my life. I wrote reams on how they had failed at this and that, and how, if they had had their acts together, I would have been born with the chance at the happiness I deserved. I denigrated them on paper, all in a supervised effort to dig up the past in order to discard it and get happy. I was still unhappy.

I was also a few other things. I was superior to the "unenlightened." I was selfish; temperamental; negative; tired and cranky. I sowed seeds of discord wherever I went. These sound suspiciously like some of the fruits of the self the Bible mentions: adultery, fornication, uncleanness, lewdness, idolatry, sorcery, hatred, contentions, outbursts of wrath, jealousies, selfish ambitions, dissensions, heresies, envy, murders, drunkenness, revelries and the like.

The Bible says, "Whatever things are true, noble, just, pure, lovely, of good report—think on these things." The Bible also says, "Honor your father and mother that your days may be long" and "He who curses father or mother, let him be put to death." It doesn't mess around with how we are to treat our parents, and there is no escape clause about "only if they did right by you." One of my biggest regrets is putting my parents through that garbage.

Using my therapy as a springboard, I eagerly catapulted headlong into the world of energy, chakras, healings, crystals, guides, pendulums, love plasma, psychic surgery and a host of other exciting, tangible examples of spiritual power. The alluring thing about all this New Age stuff was that it promised to place the power in my hands. What power was this? Control over my own life. Control, possibly even over the lives of those close to me! Too much to resist!

During therapy I developed an increasing disregard and outright scorn for what I referred to as "fundamental" Christians. I looked down my nose at my best friend because she stubbornly stuck to her "outmoded" brand of Christianity while I was cresting the wave of "cool, enlightened" Christians. I followed the advice of the ungodly, and before I knew it, I was hanging out in the halls of New Age wisdom. From there it was natural to begin to scorn "fundamental" Christians.

At the same time, in therapy I was told that the Apostle Paul was obviously a woman-hating homosexual and I believed it. How important it is for each believer to be in the Word for himself and not just assume someone is right because of his credentials, i.e., man's measurement of man.

The Bible says, "Blessed is the man who walks not in the counsel of the ungodly...." So much for my therapy. That same Psalm goes on to say, "nor standeth in the way of sinners (hangs out where temptation is) nor sitteth in the seat of the scornful." The Bible also promises, "In Jesus Christ we have redemption through His blood, the forgiveness of sins, according to the riches of His grace...." and, "Blessed are those whose lawless deeds are forgiven, and whose sins are covered; Blessed is the man to whom the Lord shall not impute sin."

For years I walked around under an enormous cloud of guilt for not being good enough. There are two ways to remedy this in my way of thinking: (A) Don't be guilty of anything, ever; or (B) Accept God's blanket pardon through acceptance of Jesus Christ as personal Lord and Savior.

I thought that enough therapy and self-help could net me the (A) result. The (A) result catered to my pride. If I tried enough, under my own power, I could become blameless. But it didn't work.

The (B) result requires acknowledging that I am unable to help myself! I have tried route (B) and have found deliverance. I don't hate my spouse anymore. I don't call my children foul names. I have merely to breathe the name of Christ and I instantly have an audience with the Maker of heaven and earth, the Creator of the universe, Almighty, Omnipotent, Omnipresent, Omniscient God. He "spreads out his ear" and listens to everything I have to say—the worthwhile and the trite. He *answers my prayers and patiently instructs, chastens, prunes and restores me in his timing and in his way.*

All this has come about since I renounced my involvement with the therapy I underwent at the hands of John French, and recanted all that garbage I had chosen to believe so that I could control my own life and be superior to everyone whom I felt threatened by because I realized if they knew me, they wouldn't like me very much.

I believe that my therapy was of the evil one, was false, was imitation salvation. Lots of Scripture was quoted but "Wisdom from above is first of all pure...." If I have to cull through a lot of dispensed "wisdom" and lean on my own understanding to pick and choose what sounds okay, it is not good. If the Bible doesn't back it up, it is not okay. Ditto the healing and its attendant trappings. It all sounded good for awhile, but it never did cure what ailed me. Sin was what ailed me. No amount of therapy can redeem our lives from the pit. Self-help is no help at all.

One last point. Therapy usually focuses on the past. Everything rotten about one's past must be dug up and faced in order to expunge it and get on with a crystal clear future. What I found is that I became mired in it. Encouraged to "go with my feelings," I wrote and wrote and WROTE and it was all foul, rotten stuff. The Bible espouses faith. Faith is choosing to believe God's Word despite feelings. Feelings are fickle and temporary; God's Word is absolute. Letting feelings rule in the place of faith is the silliest thing I have ever done.

The humiliating thing is, I believed what I was doing was right—the most superior and best form of right. All those who weren't on similar paths were stupid. I gave everyone I know, even slightly, lots of advice I had no right to give regarding this stuff. I wrote notes to newlyweds full of what I now consider poisonous advice. I pray no one took me seriously. Thank God, there was such obvious lack of good fruit in my life that people probably discounted everything I said.

In contrast, I offer a poem written one year earlier by Danita about her therapy.

> I hate the sad depressions
>   which confine me in their grip.
> I dread each lonely, painful
>   and obligatory trip.
> Is gladness so precarious
>   I lose it if I slip?
> And what of peace, that longed-for peace?
>   It seems like such a gyp.
>
> And if, in my own power,
>   I can choose to quell these spells,
> And master them with my best self,
>   as psycho-logic tells,
> Why do I feel so often
>   that I'm in a maze of hells?
> Is it self-inflicted torture,
>   'til my guilt the pain dispels?
>
> I feel so angry at the God
>   and at the man who made
> These silly rules which all us fools
>   have tried and disobeyed.
> Why set us up for failure?
>   Why assure our faults displayed?
> I think of all my wasted years.
>   I know I've been betrayed.
>
> The image set before me,
>   of perfection to attain
> Was just a false projection.

The Turning of the Tide

There was no way I could gain
Assurance of approval,
    however I might strain.
Contortions all for naught,
    I find, and all I've reaped is pain.

How could I hope to mold myself
    into what is not real?
How could I not be what I am
    and not feel what I feel?
How could I squelch the gift of God
    and try to strike a deal?
I sold out for the false
    which meant the truth I must conceal.

We all want to be loveable;
    we all want to be "good."
We attempt a transformation
    to be what we think we should.
We build our selves upon a false
    foundation made of wood.
And struggle to maintain these selves
    —as though we think we could!

We cannot maintain falsehood,
    for the yoke cannot be borne.
It's painful and degrading
    and it always leaves us torn.
We cannot with a cloak of lies
    the naked truth adorn.
We cater to our vanity,
    and God's sweet yoke we scorn.

I wonder...that betrayal
    which I bask in when I'm down...
Is it my own betrayal?
    Trading falsehood for a crown?

CHAPTER TWENTY-ONE

If an Accusation Is Made . . .

Therapies which breed the recovery of repressed memories bear remarkable similarities in methodology. Because of these similarities, and because so many families are experiencing or will experience the tragedy our family has suffered, I am going to be so bold as to offer some advice. I believe this is a crisis for which a family can easily and inexpensively prepare, and one which they can possibly avert.

I am not an expert. I have neither earned nor been honored with titles or degrees. My credentials come through the proverbial School of Hard Knocks, the "been there, done that" variety. Although my knowledge does not come from books and workshops, I have added to my personal experience by collecting and devouring as much material and information as I have found available and affordable.

With the above statement acknowledged between us, I offer some tidbits of wisdom I have accumulated along the way. The worth of these tidbits may be determined by the reader, to be heeded or discarded as you choose. I share them in the hope that they will make someone else's journey through the morass of recovered repressed memories a little less painful and a great deal less lonely than mine has been.

- If ever an accusation of sexual abuse is made within your family, immediately involve every healthy, intelligent adult family member in the situation, including those who would rather not deal with it. Resist the temptation to "shelter" the accused and to think that the less known, the better. Whether you are dealing with actual sexual abuse committed within the home or false accusations of sexual abuse hatched in a therapist's office, both thrive under cover of secrecy. Shine all the light you can on the situation. The more facts you can obtain, the better equipped you will be to make good decisions. And you will have to make decisions.
- Never, never, NEVER allow yourself or an accused loved one to "confess" to something that the accused could not remember before an accusation was made. "Repressed memories" would be more accurately described if they were called "Hellucinations Unlimited." If you didn't remember them without outside help, they are not memories!
- Chronicle the events as they happen, or as soon afterwards as possible. I believe that writing this manuscript is possibly the most significant and effective thing I have done regarding our experience, both for myself and for my entire family. Had I done it sooner, it may have brought at least partial healing to my family sooner.
- In obedience to the Biblical command to "honor thy father and mother," do not tolerate derogatory, inflammatory remarks to continually be made about your parents in your presence without refutation if you know the remarks to be untrue.
- As soon as a false accusation is made, contact the *False Memory Syndrome Foundation*. Had I had access to the kind of information and support they give, I would not have

If an Accusation Is Made . . .

stumbled around alone in the dark, and I would have known better how to proceed.
- If a case of recovered repressed memories of sexual abuse happens in your family and you know the accusations to be false, say so. Say it quickly, say it loudly and say it often. Say it to, and in the presence of, the accused. Remember, the accused stands in jeopardy of losing everything he holds near and dear, even if he is totally innocent. He has a legal right to be considered innocent until proven guilty, but that right is seldom given once an accusation of sexual abuse is made. Do not allow him to stand alone!
- If you don't know the truth, do not assume the allegation to be either true or false. Investigate and search out the truth as quickly as you can—for your sake and for the sake of every member of your extended family. Accusations become entrenched and flourish in the environment of mystery and confusion they produce. Therapists are not all-knowing gods, in spite of what they may think. It is no crime to challenge them and repudiate what they say.
- Even if you are sure you know the truth, investigate and substantiate! There should be some kind of corroborating empirical evidence of guilt, or some confirming indications of innocence. Do your best to find them. Never accept the unsubstantiated word of accuser(s) and therapists. It is usually difficult to substantiate the truth, but remember, the accuser and the therapist are counting on that fact! In one instance I know of, records proved the accused father was in Vietnam the entire period of time his daughter had indicated he had abused her! Undaunted, she and her therapist changed the charge to her uncle instead!
- If you find no evidence, insist that the accusers either produce some, or that they shut up! The American Medical Association's Council on Scientific Affairs issued the following statement dated June 16, 1994:

> *"The AMA considers recovered memories of childhood sexual abuse to be of uncertain authenticity, which should*

> be subject to external verification. The use of recovered memories is fraught with problems of potential misapplication."

- Do not fool yourself. Neutrality is a myth and a misnomer. To watch from the sidelines and do nothing while a mugger or rapist commits an act of violence against a victim is not neutrality. It is apathetic consent and constitutes aiding and abetting the perpetrator. The same is true when an accuser ravages an innocent person's reputation, destroys his life, robs him of his credibility and demolishes his personal relationships. There are no "conscientious objectors" in a false memory battle; only soldiers and cowardly defectors. Don't take my word for it. Ask anyone that has been accused if he believes his loved ones can remain neutral concerning his guilt.
- Know what is out there. What you don't know most certainly can hurt you. Therapists believe that more than 50% of American females are sexually abused. Some estimates go much higher. In many cases, the fact that your child seeks out a therapist suggests to that therapist there has been sexual abuse. Before your child opens her mouth or fills out a form, you—the parent—are often suspected of sexually abusing that child. You are already in trouble.
- Know that there is no way your child, or you, or any member of your family can convince a therapist that his or her (the therapist's) conclusions are wrong. I know of therapists who boast, "I can tell by looking at a person if they have been sexually abused." They are arrogant in their opinions of themselves and their abilities. Anyone who disagrees with them is considered ignorant, or in denial. End of subject.
- No matter what your child perceives her problem to be, some therapists believe that his or her problem stems from sexual abuse and will relentlessly push your child in that direction. Sooner or later, usually with props such as re-

quired reading, medication and/or hypnosis, the client is forced to "try to remember some occasion that could be interpreted to indicate an opportunity when abuse could have occurred." And that is all it takes. You're done.
- Upon questioning, if your child initially fails to come up with bad memories, she may be counselled that she has obviously repressed something awful which must be remembered if she is to become well. You're doomed.
- If your child succeeds in coming up with something, you're dead!
- Upon questioning, if your child thinks there might be a possibility she or he is a victim of sexual exploitation—and remember, the therapist won't accept no for an answer—that possibility translates to a "fact" etched on tablets of stone. No proof or verification is needed or wanted. You are marked.
- Upon questioning, if your child denies that she or he is a victim of sexual exploitation, that is considered an even stronger indication that it happened. In our culture, "denial" is the expected response to abuse. To the therapist, denial does not mean the event did not happen. It means the client is "in denial" of what actually did happen. You are suspect.
- Finally, upon questioning, if your child is unsure of whether she or he has been a victim of sexual abuse, that is just another indication that it happened. Being unsure is every bit as suspect as being too sure it didn't happen. You are presumed guilty.
- By now if you are under the impression that it's a "damned if you do, damned if you don't" situation, you are beginning to understand your precarious position as the parent of a son or daughter in therapy.
- Do not expect your child's therapist to be logical, reasonable, or in any way sympathetic toward you, the parent. It is almost guaranteed he will not be. You are the enemy. You should expect to be treated with scorn, disgust and hostil-

ity. Many therapists have an agenda to expose, discredit and punish you. If it later becomes apparent that you were falsely accused and that you did not sexually abuse your child, don't expect so much as a flick of an eyebrow from the accusing therapist. He couldn't care less! What is important to him is that he detected something about your child that indicated to him that abuse had occurred. That alone proves to him you are an inadequate parent.

- Just because the therapist advertises that he or she is a Christian therapist does not mean the above information does not apply or that you need not be wary. If it is important to you to have a Christian therapist, there should be evidence beyond his own declaration that the therapist is what he claims to be. Find out if he worships in a Bible-believing fellowship and talk to his pastor. Is he actively involved in a local body of believers? Do the people of his fellowship have confidence in his walk with the Lord? If those who know him best don't trust his brand of Christianity, it's probably not worth the risk to seek his counsel.
- *If you are paying for therapy for your child, your spouse or anyone else, find out what that therapist is saying about you, the payer. You could be paying the vigilante to carry out your own lynching. If you are unhappy with the therapist or the treatment he is providing, remove yourself as payer. Remember, no matter what he does "for the client's best interest," he gets big bucks for his love and concern. Cut his gravy, and he will quit dishing out the baloney! You may also notice a considerable "drying up" of the milk of human kindness.*

Scripture instructs us in Psalm 1 that *"Blessed is the man who walketh not in the counsel of the ungodly."* The entire concept of repressed memories is a colossal lie of the ungodly mind, foolishness garbed in the cloak of psychological wisdom. It exists only as a misdiagnosis of therapists or other proponents of the phenomenon and is every bit as destructive as the crime it pretends to combat—the sexual abuse of children or women. The prescribed cure—the "recovery" of repressed memories—is worse than the disease, because it requires the patient to re-live trauma that never happened in the first place.

Some people may object that there are a lot of good therapists out there, and that I have failed to mention or to recommend them. My response is that there are a lot of good parents out there that therapists generally fail to acknowledge. Our ratio of recognition is equitable.

The controversy regarding "repressed memories" is a battle for truth. Since our generation in general, and much of the psychological community in particular, has bought into the lie that truth is relative, or subjective, or "as you perceive it," these individuals can scarcely be expected to ferret out what they don't believe exists—absolute truth. Therefore, you may well find yourself alone in pursuing actual, objective, what-really-happened facts.

It is useless to seek after truth without positioning yourself on the side of truth—without having truth on your side. There is One who knows truth, who loves truth, who is Truth. If you are a person who has overlooked or rejected Him who is Truth, I recommend that you solicit his Divine guidance and intervention on your behalf.

Jesus Christ has been given the name *"Wonderful Counselor."* He remains *"our refuge and strength, a very present help in trouble,*[1]*"* and He doesn't charge huge hourly fees. If you need counseling, I heartily recommend Him. If you don't know how to receive his counsel, seek the help of a believer who is well acquainted with the Word of God and who knows how to pray.

"Blessed is the man who walketh not in the counsel of the ungodly." Be very careful where you seek counsel. I now can look back and see that the "Wonderful Counselor" of Scripture was working on our behalf even in our darkest hour. At the time I felt the most hopeless and defeated, God was moving in answer to the prayers I thought had gone unanswered. Although it took longer than I had hoped, our family is once again basically unified. Misinformation has been corrected and misunderstandings have been sorted out.

Skeletons Without Bones

What of my sister Lillian? I believe that in answer to prayer on her behalf—Daddy's included—Lillian will be brought face to face with what Francis Schaeffer called "true truth." By that he meant "what actually is fact, regardless of individual perceptions." In Lillian's case, this would mean she would finally comprehend the truth about her past, her father, herself, and her therapist. What she then chooses to do with that truth will shape her destiny.

I believe she will, after all, embrace "true truth."

EPILOGUE

Why This Book?

I have been asked why I would bother to write this book. After all, my father has been dead for a number of years. Family members are all speaking to one another in civil tones. Why would I risk the animosity that would surely follow in the wake of such a publication?

First, I owe it to my father. He went to his grave with his name degraded and his character attacked. I had vowed I would investigate the charges. I turned every rock I could find that might present a clue one way or another.

If I had found evidence that Lillian was telling the truth, I had determined I would be her advocate and champion. If she had truly suffered what she claimed, she needed and deserved as much. All of my family would have been apprised of my findings, however much it hurt—because I believe wholesome lives and meaningful relationships are possible only when they are based on truth. In the physical realm, the mental realm, and the spiritual realm, wherever falsehood or deceit exists, the foundations crumble and the superstructure collapses.

However, in turning over the boulders of our past, I stumbled onto no slime, exposed no creepy crawly things, uncovered no cesspools. Instead I found good soil, sparkling springs and a deep vein of pure gold. Everywhere I searched, priceless treasure presented itself, ready to be claimed and mined.

If I were obligated to act responsibly by exposing any undesirable secrets I might have uncovered concerning my dad, even though such news would have devastated a large number of my loved ones, then I am equally obligated to openly affirm and revel in the wholesome, moral uprightness that I discovered, though it flies in the face of the declarations of one lone accuser and her supporters.

I owe it to my father to tell what I know.

Second, I owe it to my mother. Fully alive, Mom knows that along with Dad she stands accused. I also am a mother. If ever one of my boys were to point a finger at either his father or myself in unfounded allegations, I would look confidently to the other son to counter with a defense. Imperfect parents we are, but that does not make us unconscionable perverts, preying on our innocent children. In the face of an unwarranted attack by one son, I would find the silence of the second son every bit as incomprehensible as the noise of the first. As much as to my father, I owe this book to my mother.

I owe it to my boys. They are descendants of John E. McGraw. They deserve to know from whence they have come. Had I found some sordid trail of misdeeds perpetrated by their grandfather, we would have had to acknowledge and live with it. But there is neither virtue nor glory in taking upon our backs a loathsome burden manufactured and assigned to us by some misguided guru.

I owe it to my boys to provide them with the truth about their heritage. Since the sins of the fathers are visited upon the children unto the third and fourth generation, but the deeds of the righteous to a thousand generations,[1] I want them to know that their good minds and their stalwart constitutions are benefits they enjoy at least in part because of forebears who honored God with their lives. They do not have to struggle under the shame of a curse that is not theirs to bear. I owe it to my sons and their entire generation of cousins to pass on to them the truth concerning their priceless heritage.

I owe it to my brothers and sisters. Not one of them, other than Lillian, was present in the office that morning I met with Dr. French. They had never heard the story from me in its entirety. They have been given the opportunity to read this manuscript. They can now make conclusions based on full disclosure rather than on ugly bits and pieces pasted together in some sort of dreadful collage.

I owe it to my two sisters most affected, Ginny and Lillian. They have been left a legacy by each of two men who shared a common name. They had been mistaken about the nature and value of these very different legacies. One John prayed for them. The other John preyed upon them. I owe them the truth. I love them enough to risk telling them the truth. I have given both Lillian and Ginny a copy of this manuscript. Perhaps their responses will provide material for a sequel!

I owe it to a multitude of people who find themselves in a situation similar to ours. A few of them I have met. Most of them I will never know. These are the more than twenty thousand families who within the first five and one-half years of its existence have made contact with the *False Memory Syndrome Foundation* because they too have been dragged into the same stinking pit in which we find ourselves. They too gag and choke on sewage not their own.

It is often said that "misery loves company." This particular misery finds in fellow sufferers a veritable lifeline to which they cling as they strive to keep their heads above the morass. Some dare not speak. Some have spoken only to find that no one listens. Others cannot speak; they only weep.

I owe it to these, my fellows, to speak to an awakening world. If I can reach even a small audience, perhaps some will rise up and say, "Enough! Away with these licensed saboteurs educated beyond their knowledge who, professing themselves to be wise, have become fools."[2]

I owe it to all who tragically and actually have been abused. Rather than seeking to unearth torturous memories, these people have been unable to forget what happened to them. They have had to live every day of their lives with memories they gladly would have forgotten if they could have done so.[3]

These are true victims. They should be able to tell their stories without having to compete with the lurid details of trumped-up violations by sadistic-minded attention-seekers. They should be able to find listening, sympathetic ears that have not been jaded and de-sensitized by oft-repeated myths and fables of those whose memories have only recently begun to serve them as a result of therapy, suggestion or hypnosis.

But mostly, I wrote it for Daddy.

Notes

Chapter One

[1] Throughout this book names have been changed unless permission to use actual names has been granted.
[2] Registered Trademark, Parker Brothers.
[3] *Radio Talks for Children*, author and publisher unknown.

Chapter Two

[1] At the time I wrote this in 1977, I thought Lillian's accusations were limited to her perception that Mother and Daddy never wanted her, never loved her, and similar complaints. I considered her charges unfounded and nearly blasphemous at the time, though they were bland compared to later charges. I had no clue sexual allegations and other distortions would later come to light. Though my knowledge was limited, my outrage was complete.
[2] Registered trademark.
[3] Author unknown, "The Bremen-Town Musicians," *Favorite Stories* (Western Publishing, 1944, 1966), pp. 14-17.
[4] Joseph Bert Smiley, *St. Peter at the Gate*. This poem originally appeared in the Brooklyn *Eagle* titled *Thirty Years with a Shrew*, date unknown.

Skeletons Without Bones

[5] Will Carleton, *Caleb's Courtship*.
[6] I Wish You Had Known **My** Daddy - Donna M. Laurence, 1977, Revised 1994.

Chapter Three

[1] Arthur Janov, *The Primal Scream* (Perigee, 1970).
[2] See Richard Ofshe and Ethan Watters, "Making Monsters," *Society*, March/April 1993, p.9. Repressed memory therapists claim the first step in effecting a cure is to "get the trusting, unaware but possibly resistant, client to agree that brutalization did occur—most likely by a relative....The therapist's expectations predict the direction of the treatment."
[3] Rita L. Atkinson, et al, *Introduction to Psychology* (Harcourt Brace Jovanovich, 1987), p. 265.
[4] Cf. Richard Ofshe and Ethan Watters, op.cit., p.5. The term repression "has been used in different ways in the mental health community for 100 years. Freud employed the term to describe the mind's conscious and unconscious avoidance of unpleasant wishes, thoughts, or memories. Even under this conservative definition, the existence of repression has never been empirically demonstrated. Sixty years of experiments have failed to produce evidence of its existence."

Chapter Four

[1] See Hebrews 11:17-19.
[2] II Timothy 3:16, New International Version.
[3] Martin Gardner, "The False Memory Syndrome," *Skeptical Inquirer*, Summer 1993, p. 370. In Freud's early career he made extensive use of hypnotism. He "was amazed by the number of mesmerized women who dredged up childhood memories of being raped by their fathers. It was years before he became convinced that most of these women were fantasizing. Other analysts and psychiatrists agreed."
[4] "An unscrupulous therapist never lets you get over your past. The [recovered memory] movement is all about telling the patient you can never grow up and be an independent person because you are fatally flawed. The recovery movement is a marvelous money spinner because no one in the recovery movement ever recovers." Dr. Dorothy

Rowe, Clinical Psychologist in "Therapists Accused of Misleading Patients" by Rosie Waterhouse, *The Independent*, June 1, 1994 as quoted in June 1994 issue of the *False Memory Syndrome Foundation Newsletter*.

Chapter Six

[1] Luke 8:50, King James Version.
[2] At that time I thought there had to be an unknown pre-existent cause for her emotional deterioration. Now I know that drug use, hypnosis, and biased therapists are sufficient ingredients for personality deterioration, and that the abuser in Lillian's life has been her therapist.
[3] A term signifying a designated Bible teacher who would fill the pulpit in the absence of the resident pastor.

Chapter Eight

[1] 1 *Cheaper by the Dozen*, Evangeline Gilbert
[2] See Numbers 22:28-30.
[3] Elizabeth Loftus and Katherine Ketcham, *Witness for the Defense* (St. Martins Press, 1991), p.231.

Chapter Eleven

[1] Pamela Freyd, *False Memory Syndrome Foundation Newsletter*, April 1994, p.1. "We do not have to say that they [those in opposition to the FMS debate] are hiding or inventing evidence. Quite the contrary. What we are saying is that they seem not to care about evidence."

Chapter Thirteen

[1] John Taylor, "The Lost Daughter," *Esquire*, March 1994, pp.84,85. "Hypnotized patients will just as easily accept premises that contradict their core convictions and actual experiences as they will those that reflect them. Memories can be vivid under hypnosis...but they aren't necessarily true (Spiegel)."

Chapter Sixteen

[1] Ronald Salafia quoted in "Science or Belief Systems," *False Memory Syndrome Foundation Newsletter*, March 1994, p.2. "Memories from infancy are highly suspect at best. Normally, no one has memories until at least two or three and sometimes three or four. Before that memories are not stored in a fashion that's retrievable."

Chapter Eighteen

[1] M. Horn, "Memories Lost and Found," *U.S. News and World Report*, Nov. 29, 1993, p. 56. Patients "may embrace a 'discovery' of past abuse because it offers a single, unambiguous explanation for complex problems and a special identity as 'survivors'."

[2] I do not know when Lillian changed the age at which her alleged abuse had occurred. The letter mentioned above stating "3 or 4 or 5" was written in 1980. In 1993, in the presence of three nieces, Anna and myself, she said she was about 18 months old at the time of the abuse.

[3] This alludes to Lillian being the ninth occupant of a three-room house!

[4] The opinions expressed here are not necessarily those of the author— nor of a certain missionary I know!

[5] Mrs. Scott mentioned leaving Mark with us while they went to Haiti; Lillian mentions their second child, Starr. I believe we kept them both.

[6] Common over-the-counter drugs such as aspirin, as well as certain prescribed medications.

Chapter Ninteen

[1] False Memory Syndrome Foundation, 3401 Market Street-Suite 130, Philadelphia, Pennsylvania 19104-3315, Pamela Freyd, Ph. D. Executive Director.

[2] Cf. Martin Gardner, op. cit., p. 374. Repressed memory therapists "deny asking leading questions but tapes of their sessions often prove otherwise. If no memories surface, they will prod a patient to make up a story. After many repetitions and elaborations of the invented scenario, the patient starts to believe the story is true."

[3] See Lawrence Wright, *Remembering Satan* (Alfred A. Knopf, 1994), pp.35, 194.

Chapter Twenty

[1] Pam Forster, *For Instruction in Righteousness* (1993).

Chapter Twenty-One

[1] Psalm 46:1, King James Version.

Epilogue

[1] See Exodus 20:4, Commandment #2 of the Ten Commandments.
[2] See Romans 1:22, King James Version, the words of St. Paul.
[3] Cf. M. Horn, op. cit., p.55. Psychiatry professor Paul McHugh of John Hopkins University says, "Most severe traumas are not blocked out by children but remembered all too well."

Bibliography

Almy, Gary and Almy, Carol Tharp. *Addicted to Recovery*. Eugene, Oregon: Harvest House Publishers, 1994.

Bulkley, Ed. *Why Christians Can't Trust Psychology*. Eugene, Oregon: Harvest House Publishers, 1993.

Freyd, Pamela and Goldstein, Eleanor. *Smiling Through Tears*. Boca Raton, Florida: Upton Books (SIRS), 1997.

Ganz, Richard. *Psychobabble*. Wheaton, Illinois: Crossway Books, 1993.

Goldstein, Eleanor and Farmer, Kevin. *True Stories of False Memories*. Boca Raton, Florida: SIRS Books, 1993.

Hunt, Dave and McMahon, T.A. *The Seduction of Christianity*. Eugene, Oregon: Harvest House Publishers, 1985.

Idomir, Louise S. *Psychology: Pied Piper of New Age*. Hearthstone Publishing, Ltd.

Kilpatrick, William Kirk. *Psychological Seduction*. New York: Thomas Nelson Publishers, 1983.

Loftus, Elizabeth and Ketcham, Katherine. *The Myth of Repressed Memory*. New York: St. Martin's Press, 1991.

Ofshe, Richard and Watters, Ethan. *Making Monsters*. New York: Schribners, 1994.

Owen, Jim. *Christian Psychology's War on God's Word*. Santa Barbara: EastGate Publishers, 1993.

Wright, Lawrence. *Remembering Satan*. New York: Knopf, 1994.

To order additional copies of:

Skeletons Without Bones

send $15.95 plus $3.95 shipping and handling to:

WinePress Publishing
PO Box 1406
Mukilteo, WA 98275

or have your credit card ready and call:

(800) 917-BOOK